Control irritable bowel syndrome for life

IBS
FOOD, FACTS
& RECIPES

TRACY PARKER & SARA LEWIS

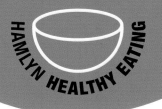

HAMLYN HEALTHY EATING

An Hachette UK company
www.hachette.co.uk

First published in Great Britain in 2007 by
Hamlyn, a division of Octopus Publishing Group Limited
Endeavour House, 189 Shaftesbury Avenue,
London WC2H 8JY
www.octopusbooksusa.com

This edition published in 2015

Distributed in the US by Hachette Book Group
1290 Avenue of the Americas, 4th and 5th Floors
New York, NY 10020

Distributed in Canada by Canadian Manda Group
664 Annette Street, Toronto, Ontario, Canada M6S 2C8

Tracy Parker and Sara Lewis assert the moral right to be
identified as the authors of this work.

ISBN 978-0600-63081-4

Printed and bound in China

10 9 8 7 6 5 4 3 2 1

Nutritional analysis is provided for each recipe and given
per serving.

People with known nut allergies should avoid recipes
containing nuts or nut derivatives, and vulnerable people
should avoid dishes containing raw or lightly cooked eggs.

If you are avoiding wheat and gluten, double-check the
ingredients list on items such as mustard and bouillon
cubes before use. In addition, some brands of cornstarch
contain wheat flour to keep it free flowing, so read the
ingredients list carefully if you are avoiding gluten.

Many of the recipes can be adapted for either a high- or
low-fiber diet by using brown or white rice, pasta, and flour
or by using different combinations of vegetables, and
recipes can be adapted for milk-free diets by the inclusion
of soy milk and yogurt instead of cows' milk and yogurt.

Part of the nutritional information provided is sodium.
These amounts only cover added salt when a specific
amount is stated in the recipes.

contents

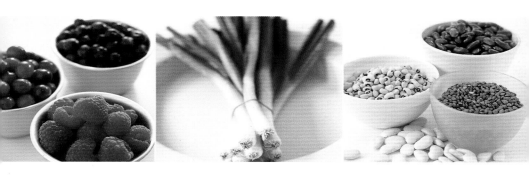

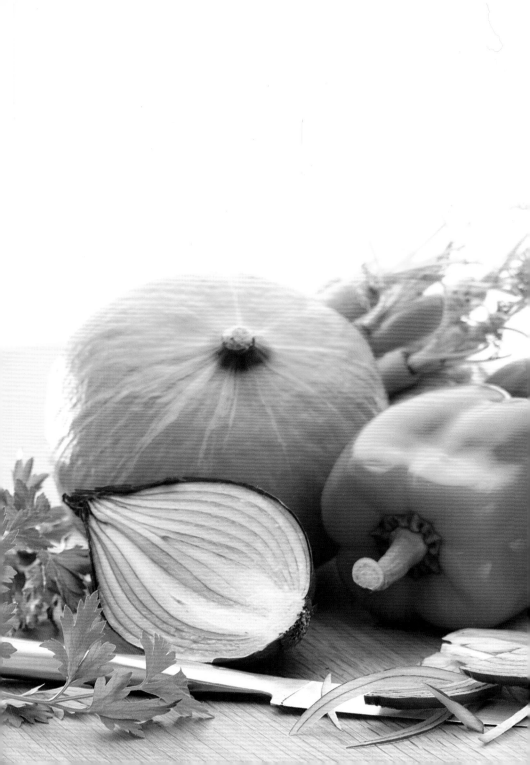

introduction

Irritable Bowel Syndrome (IBS) is a common bowel condition, which is said to affect as many as one in five of the adult populations of Britain and the USA. People of any age can suffer with IBS, including children, but the most common age range affected is 20–40 years, and women are twice as likely to report symptoms of IBS than men.

The cause of IBS is not known, although there are many factors involved, and often the symptoms are the result of a combination of factors rather than just one. At present, there is no single cure for IBS, but there are lots of different ways to manage it, and tailoring your diet to deal with the symptoms you experience is a good place to start. It is important to remember, however, that dietary changes will not help everyone, and if your symptoms persist you should seek medical advice.

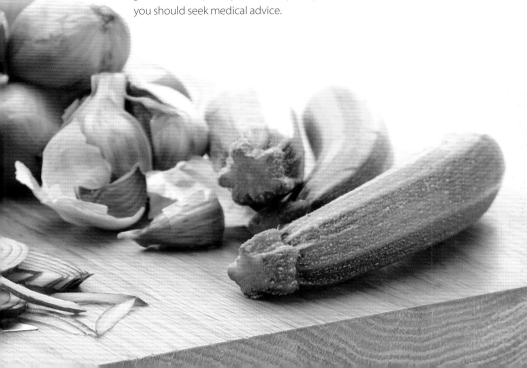

what is Irritable Bowel Syndrome?

"Self-diagnosis of IBS is not advisable. Before a diagnosis is made it is important that a doctor carries out appropriate examinations and investigations."

Irritable Bowel Syndrome (IBS) is described as a functional bowel disorder by the medical profession. This means that no specific cause can be found for an individual's symptoms after medical investigations but that the bowel is functioning in an abnormal way.

Symptoms

The key symptoms for a diagnosis of IBS are that the person should have suffered abdominal pain or discomfort for at least 12 weeks (this does not have to be consecutive weeks) during the last 12 months. In addition, two of the following three symptoms should also be present:

- ☐ Relief of pain or discomfort with passing a bowel motion (defecation)
- ☐ A change in the frequency of stools—an increase or decrease in bowel motions
- ☐ A change in the consistency of stools—looser or harder motions

Additional symptoms

There is a further group of symptoms that support the diagnosis of IBS, and two or more of these should be present on at least 25 percent of occasions or days when IBS is suspected. These supportive symptoms are:

- ☐ Altered stool frequency: more than three bowel motions a day or fewer than three bowel movements a week
- ☐ Altered stool form: looser or more watery motions, or hard, lumpy or pellet-like motions
- ☐ Altered stool passage: straining to pass a motion or urgency or the feeling of not completely emptying the bowel (incomplete evacuation)

OTHER CONDITIONS WITH SIMILAR SYMPTOMS

- Diverticulitis
- Gallstones
- Bile salt malabsorption
- Microscopic colitis
- Chronic fatigue syndrome
- Celiac disease
- Inflammatory bowel disease (Crohn's disease or ulcerative colitis)
- Bowel cancer

□ Passing mucus with stools
□ Abdominal bloating or distension

In addition to the above symptoms, many people with IBS often complain of flatulence (wind), rumbling noises in the bowel (borborygmi), indigestion or heartburn, nausea, headaches, persistent tiredness, and an increased need to urinate. Women sometimes also find sexual intercourse painful.

Is it IBS?

Self-diagnosis of IBS is not advisable. Before a diagnosis is made it is important that a medical doctor carries out appropriate examinations and investigations. This is because there are several other, more serious bowel conditions that have similar symptoms to those of IBS. Further investigation may be necessary if any of the following are present:

□ Recent, unexplained weight loss
□ Rectal bleeding
□ Anemia
□ Fever
□ Start of symptoms over the age of 50 years
□ Recurrent vomiting
□ A family history of colon cancer, Crohn's disease, ulcerative colitis, or celiac disease

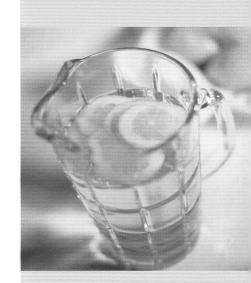

possible causes of IBS

"It is not known if stress causes IBS in the first place, but the symptoms of IBS can certainly make people anxious."

There are many different theories about the causes of IBS, and there are almost as many different ideas about how to treat it. The main causes are believed to be a bout of bacterial gastroenteritis, the use of antibiotics, stress and anxiety and other psychological reasons, abnormal gut motility and hypersensitivity of the gut, the menstrual cycle in women, and diet.

Post-infective IBS

Some people with IBS can link the start of their symptoms to having had a bowel infection or gastroenteritis, such as salmonella food poisoning. Research has shown that people who have had severe gastroenteritis are almost 12 times more likely to develop IBS than those who have not. It is not clear why this is the case, although changes to a person's normal gut bacteria have been suggested, as have slight changes to the bowel itself. This type of IBS is known as post-infective IBS.

Antibiotics

Everyone's large bowel contains billions of bacteria. The bacteria are of hundreds of different types, some of them beneficial to our health and others with the potential to cause ill health. In normal circumstances these bacteria live in a balance together and cause no problems to the individual. However, a course of antibiotics, prescribed to kill the bacteria causing a particular infection, can also kill the good bacteria in the bowel. This leads to an imbalance, which can result in symptoms such as diarrhea, abdominal bloating, pain, and flatulence.

Stress and anxiety

Many people find that stress or anxiety triggers their IBS, and some sufferers can link the start of their symptoms with times of change or upheaval in their life, such as leaving home, starting work, getting married, or going to university. Other upsetting events include relationship problems, bereavement, and physical or sexual abuse.

Stress has been shown to increase the speed at which waste is moved through the large bowel (colon), so leading to more frequent bowel motions. It also releases chemicals in the body that stimulate the colon, which leads to pain. It is not known if stress causes IBS in the first place, but the symptoms of IBS can certainly make people anxious, especially if their symptoms are frequent and unpleasant. Some people with IBS also have psychiatric illnesses.

Abnormal gut movement and hypersensitivity

Research has shown that in some people with IBS waste is moved through the gut more slowly or more quickly than normal. A slower movement may result in constipation, whereas a faster movement may lead to diarrhea. There is also evidence that some people with IBS are more sensitive to discomfort in the bowel than people without IBS.

Research is being carried out into the ways in which the brain deals with pain or the anticipation of pain because there is some evidence that this does not work normally in IBS sufferers.

Menstrual cycle

IBS symptoms can be affected by the change in hormone levels that occur in the body over the menstrual cycle. Most women notice a change in their bowel motions during menstruation. It is not more common in IBS, but it may have more effect. As with some menstrual disorders, evening primrose oil may help with IBS symptoms.

"Exercise stimulates the body to produce feel good substances called endorphines, which help reduce stress."

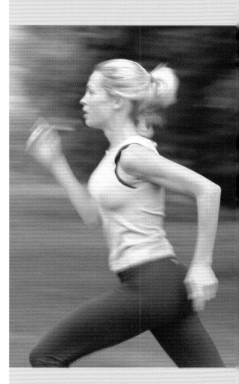

diet and IBS

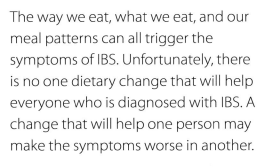

DIETARY FACTORS LINKED WITH IBS

- Meal pattern
- Fluid intake
- Dietary fiber intake
- Food intolerance
- Irritants to the bowel, such as caffeine, alcohol, and spicy foods
- Abnormal digestion of lactose and fructose
- Fatty foods
- Excessive intake of intestinal stimulants, such as sorbitol

The way we eat, what we eat, and our meal patterns can all trigger the symptoms of IBS. Unfortunately, there is no one dietary change that will help everyone who is diagnosed with IBS. A change that will help one person may make the symptoms worse in another.

Meal patterns

It is important to have regular meals throughout the day. Missing meals and then snacking on high-fat, sugary foods or having one huge meal a day can lead to bloating, abdominal discomfort, and wind.

How and what we eat

Eating quickly and rushing meals can lead to air being swallowed at the same time. This can result in belching or indigestion, and it can cause abdominal bloating and wind. Eating slumped over a computer keyboard or dashing around at the same time as eating can also cause problems. Always take time over your meals and sit up straight when you are eating.

Many foods have been identified as triggers to IBS symptoms, and these are considered in more detail on the following pages. However, simply adopting a balanced diet quite often helps people with IBS to control their symptoms.

Portion sizes

The bowel is made up of muscles that contract and relax one after another in sequence to push food through the digestive tract. A large meal can cause a stronger wave of muscle contraction, resulting in abdominal discomfort, indigestion, and nausea. Keep to moderate portion sizes and healthy eating guidelines.

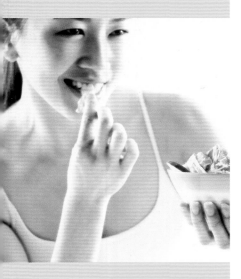

a balanced diet

A balanced diet is one that provides the body with all the nutrients it requires for health. In practice, this means choosing foods from the five food groups in the recommended amounts. The five food groups are: proteins, starchy foods, milk and dairy products, fruit and vegetables, and fats and sugars.

Protein

The body needs protein for growth and to repair cells. Protein-containing foods can be divided into animal proteins and vegetable proteins. Animal sources of protein are meat, including poultry and variety meats, fish, and eggs; vegetable sources are beans, lentils, and nuts. These foods are also good sources of iron, zinc, magnesium, and B vitamins.

It is recommended that we include two servings of these foods a day. Try to choose leaner cuts of meat, trim away visible fat and remove the skin from poultry. You should also avoid frying meat to keep your fat intake down. This is recommended for general health, but fatty foods can also make IBS symptoms worse.

Starchy foods

Starchy foods are good sources of carbohydrates, which provide energy as well as B vitamins and fiber. Bread, pasta, rice, breakfast cereals, and potatoes are good sources of starchy carbohydrates, and it is recommended that one-third of our daily diet should come from these foods—around 7–10 portions a day for women and 8–12 portions a day for men—so including a starchy food at every meal is important.

GUIDELINE PORTIONS OF PROTEIN FOODS

3½ oz lean meat or poultry

3½ oz oily fish

5 oz white fish

2 eggs

4 tablespoons of cooked legumes or lentils

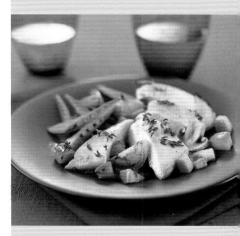

GUIDELINE PORTIONS OF STARCHY FOODS

1 slice of medium-cut bread

½ roll

½ pita bread

1 small chapatti

2 egg-sized potatoes

2 heaped tablespoons of cooked rice or pasta

3 crispbreads or crackers

3 tablespoons of breakfast cereal

3 tablespoons of rolled oats

GUIDELINE PORTIONS OF MILK AND DAIRY PRODUCTS

1½ oz cheese

¾ cup milk

½ cup yogurt

¾ cup calcium-enriched soy milk

¾ cup calcium-enriched rice milk

½ cup soy dessert or yogurt

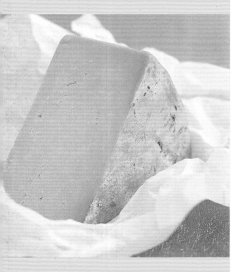

"It is recommended that no more than one-twelfth of our daily food intake comes from fats and sugars."

Milk and dairy products

Milk and dairy products are an excellent source of calcium, as well as protein and vitamins A, B12, and D. Included in this group are milk, cheese and yogurt. Butter and cream are not included because they are high in fat and are therefore found in the fats and sugar group. It is recommended that we include three servings of these foods a day.

Fruit and vegetables

Fruit and vegetables are good sources of vitamin C, folate, carotenoids, potassium, and fiber. All types of fruit and vegetable are included in this group except potatoes, which are classed as a starchy food. Fruit and vegetables can be fresh, frozen, canned, or dried. It is recommended that we have a minimum of five portions of these foods each day (see page 17).

Fats and sugars

Fatty and sugary foods tend to be high in calories and low in essential nutrients, and are often high in salt. Although it is fine to include them in small amounts in a varied diet, too much of them can lead to weight gain. It is recommended that only one-twelfth of our daily food intake comes from these foods. High-fat foods include butter, margarine, oils, fried foods, chips and savory snacks, and pastry. High-sugar foods include candy, chocolate, cakes, cookies, soft drinks and drinks, and ice cream.

How much fluid?

It is recommended that we have 6–8 cups of fluid a day, which is equivalent to 3–4 pints. It is a myth that this fluid should be made up of just water. Any type of drink counts toward the recommended amount (except alcohol). Certain types of drinks, however, can trigger symptoms of IBS (see page 13).

Fluids

As much as 70 percent of an adult's body weight is water. Throughout the day we lose water in our sweat, breath, urine, and feces, and if we do not replace the fluid we lose we suffer from dehydration, which leads to headaches, a lack of concentration, tiredness, and dark-colored urine. Continued inadequate intakes can lead to constipation and increase the risk of cystitis.

There are times when your body will need more fluid, such as when exercising, in a hot environment, if you have a temperature, or if you have frequent diarrhea or vomiting.

Caffeine As a stimulant caffeine gives us the kick-start we sometimes need. However, it also acts as an irritant to the bowel and can increase the need to urinate. Excessive amounts of caffeine can exacerbate the symptoms of IBS, so keep to a maximum of four or five caffeine-rich drinks a day and alternate them with caffeine-free drinks or water. Remember that some foods and pain-killing tablets contain caffeine too.

Alcohol Alcohol is also an irritant to the bowel and it can contribute to diarrhea, abdominal discomfort, and indigestion (heartburn). Ideally, keep within the recommended sensible limits for alcohol (around 14 units a week for women and 21 units a week for men) and have some alcohol-free days. Alcohol does help us to relax, and stress is linked with IBS, so a glass of wine at the end of a busy day can be helpful.

Carbonated drinks The gas in carbonated drinks can give abdominal bloating, belching, and discomfort. Limit your intake of these drinks to one glass of 1–1¼ cups (8–10 oz) a day. These drinks include sparkling water, lemonade, cola, mixers added to spirits, soda water, and sparkling fruit juice drinks.

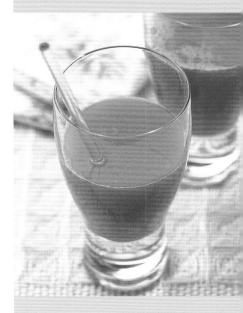

CAFFEINE-RICH FOODS AND DRINKS

- Coffee, tea, hot chocolate, performance drinks, cola, and chocolate

CAFFEINE-FREE DRINKS

- Decaffeinated coffee and tea, milk and soy milk, herbal and fruit teas, fruit juice, fruit concentrates, still mineral water and flavored still water, tapwater

ALCOHOL UNITS

For the purposes of assessing your intake, one unit of alcohol is:

1 bottle (12 oz) standard-strength beer, lager, or hard cider

1 small glass (5 oz) wine

1 glass of sherry

1 shot (1½ oz) of spirits

dietary fiber

GOOD SOURCES OF SOLUBLE FIBER:

- Oats, barley, legumes, seeds, fruit and vegetables

GOOD SOURCES OF INSOLUBLE FIBER:

- Skins, peel, and seeds on fruit and vegetables, wheat, rye, and nuts

SOURCES OF RESISTANT STARCH:

- Cooked potato, pasta, and rice eaten cold or re-heated

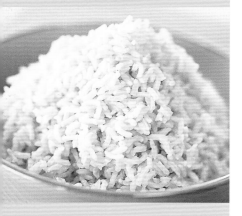

Dietary fiber, sometimes referred to as roughage, is part of plant foods that our bodies find hard to digest. It is found in fruits, vegetables, cereals, legumes, nuts and seeds. It is part of the carbohydrate family, along with sugars and starches, and is known as complex carbohydrate or non-starch polysaccharide (NSP) in the scientific world.

Bacteria

Bacteria in the large intestine are able to break down fiber by a process called fermentation. This results in the production of gases, which are removed from the body as wind or are carried by the bloodstream to the lungs and expired on the breath. They also create substances called short chain fatty acids, which provide essential energy for the cells of the large intestine and also for the growth of the bacteria themselves.

Soluble and insoluble fiber

Fiber is divided into two types: soluble and insoluble fiber. Soluble fiber forms a gel-like substance in the intestine, and it has been shown to lower blood sugar and cholesterol levels.

Insoluble fiber absorbs water and helps provide bulky, easier-to-pass stools.

Resistant starch

Starch is found in foods such as potatoes, bread, and rice and in some fruits. It was thought that all starch was digested in the small intestine, but it is now known that some starch is resistant to this process. It reaches the large intestine, where it is fermented by gut bacteria.

high and low fiber

IBS symptoms can be affected by the amount of fiber in your diet. Too little fiber can cause constipation and too much can cause bloating, discomfort, and wind. It can also trigger diarrhea. Altering the amount and type of fiber you eat can help control IBS symptoms.

High-fiber diets

A high-fiber diet may benefit people whose main symptom of IBS is constipation without abdominal bloating or wind.

It is important to increase the intake of both soluble and insoluble fiber and to have an adequate fluid intake—that is, 6–8 cups or 3–4 pints every day. Increase your intake of fiber gradually, over several days, because a sudden increase can give abdominal discomfort and wind. In addition, there is no benefit from having more than about 1 oz of fiber a day, and the recommended daily intake is just over ½ oz.

Fiber supplements

Adding wheat bran to the diet to increase fiber intake is not recommended. Research has shown that it can make the symptoms of abdominal pain and bloating worse, and bran also interferes with the absorption of minerals, such as calcium, zinc, and iron, from the diet.

Low-fiber diets

Healthy-eating guidelines suggest that we should increase our intake of fiber to decrease the risk of developing bowel cancer and diverticular disease. However, some people with IBS find that increasing their fiber intake makes their symptoms worse. A low-

INCREASING FIBER INTAKE

Among the best ways of increasing your intake of fiber are:

- Choosing whole-wheat, multigrain, or seeded breads
- Changing to brown rice or whole-wheat pasta or mixing half white and half brown together
- Keeping the skins on vegetables and fruit
- Eating whole-wheat breakfast cereals, such as Weetabix or bran flakes, or oat-based cereals, such as porridge
- Aiming to have at least five portions of fruit and vegetables every day
- Having seeds, nuts, or dried fruit as snacks
- Adding legumes to stews and casseroles

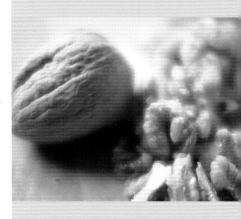

DECREASING FIBER INTAKE

Among the best ways of decreasing your intake of fiber are:

- Changing to white bread and rolls
- Choosing baked products made with white flour, such as muffins, scones, crumpets, and cake
- Having white pasta and rice and always eating it hot (cold pasta and rice are high in resistant starch)
- Avoiding the skins and peel on fruit and vegetables, including the skins on baked and new potatoes
- Limiting fruit and vegetables to a maximum of five portions a day and choosing ones from the lower-fiber list (see right)
- Eating lower-fiber breakfast cereals, such as cornflakes and rice crispies

REINTRODUCING HIGHER-FIBER FOODS

It is important to add higher-fiber foods back to the diet gradually. A sudden increase can lead to pain, wind, bloating, and diarrhea. Different people find that they can tolerate different amounts and types of fibre. Following a reintroduction program can help to identify these more easily.

Week 1 Keep skins and peel on fruit and vegetables

Week 2 Include one portion of a higher-fiber fruit or vegetable daily (see page 17); still aim for at least 5 portions a day

Week 3 Include oat products, such as porridge and oatcakes

Week 4 Change to whole-wheat bread

Week 5 Try eating wholegrain breakfast cereals

fiber diet can help people whose symptoms of IBS are either diarrhea with abdominal bloating and wind or constipation with abdominal bloating and wind.

Limiting your intake of fiber may help IBS symptoms because it will decrease the amount of bacterial fermentation that occurs in the large bowel. This will lead to less gas being produced and so reduce bloating. It will also mean that stools will be less bulky and their movement through the bowel will be slowed down.

Following a lower-fiber diet for four weeks will be long enough to know if it is going to help or not. It is a good idea to keep a record of the food and drink you take and any symptoms you experience, because it will show if there has been any improvement. If your symptoms do improve it is advisable to gradually reintroduce higher-fiber food to your diet to find a level that you can tolerate (see left).

If there has been no improvement after four weeks there is no need to remain on the diet and you should return to a normal diet.

Vegetarians and low fiber

Vegetarians who depend for their protein on legumes, lentils, nuts, and seeds will have to include small portions of these foods once a day when they are on a low-fiber diet unless other sources of protein, such as milk, cheese, eggs, and yogurt, are included at each meal.

Bulking agents and low-fiber diets

People who have a tendency to constipation should include a bulking agent, such as sterculia, psyllium husks, methylcellulose or linseeds, so that their constipation does not become worse. These agents can be obtained from health food stores and pharmacies. It is important to take them with plenty of fluid—say a generous cup—as they form a gel when eaten, which provides bulk to help stimulate a bowel motion. They should be taken every day.

Portions of fruit and vegetables

One portion of fruit is equal to 3–3½ oz or 1½ oz of dried fruit. One portion of vegetables is about 3 oz (see right). These weights refer to the edible parts only, so skins and peel of fresh produce that are not normally eaten and the juice or water of canned foods are not included in the total.

Highs and lows of fruit and vegetables

The fiber content of the fruit and vegetables listed below is based on one standard portion. Fruits and vegetables that are not included in the tables have a moderate fiber intake. These can be included in the daily diet, but keep them to one portion a day.

Higher-fiber fruit and vegetables Aduki beans, apricots (dried), baked beans, baked potato with skin, black currants, black eye beans, cabbage, cranberries, figs (dried), gooseberries, green beans, kidney beans, navy beans, and peas.

Lower-fiber fruit and vegetables Apple (peeled), apricots, bell peppers, cucumber, grapefruit, grapes, leeks, lettuce, melon, mushrooms, nectarine (peeled), onions, peaches (peeled), radishes, scallions, tomatoes, and zucchini.

GUIDE FOR ONE PORTION OF FRUIT

2 small fruits, such as fresh apricots

1 medium fruit, such as apples

1 slice of large fruit, such as melon

1 tablespoon dried fruit, such as raisins

2–3 larger dried fruits, such as dates

GUIDE FOR ONE PORTION OF VEGETABLES

3 large tablespoons cooked vegetables

Small bowl of salad

3 tablespoons beans or legumes

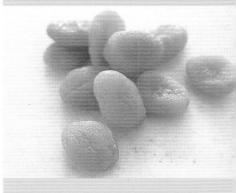

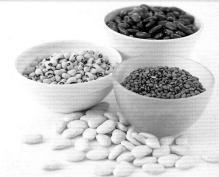

food intolerance or allergy?

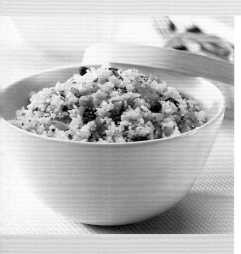

The terms food intolerance and allergy mean different things to different people. Just to confuse things even further there is also something known as food sensitivity. It is important to understand the differences between each of them.

Food allergy

An allergic response to food occurs when the body's immune system identifies a particular food as harmful to it. In response, the body produces antibodies, which can be measured by blood tests or skin prick tests. Only a small amount of the food needs to be eaten to lead to an allergic reaction. Eating the food and the appearance of symptoms can be almost immediate, but there are some conditions, such as celiac disease (see page 24), where an allergy to a food occurs much more slowly.

"It is thought that 1–2 percent of the general population have a food allergy, and the percentage is higher among children."

Food intolerance

Food intolerance does not affect the immune system, and in general the symptoms take longer to occur after eating a particular food. Often, large amounts of a food have to be eaten to trigger a response. The symptoms can be similar to those of a true food allergy—rashes, diarrhea and vomiting, for example—and for some people symptoms can be quite severe.

Testing and food intolerance

The tests used to show food allergy, such as blood tests and skin prick tests, cannot be used to identify food intolerance as it is not the result of changes in the immune system.

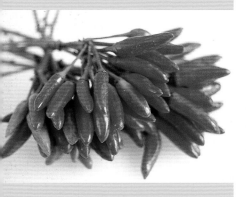

There is a wide range of tests that claim to identify food intolerance, such as hair testing, pulse testing, and measuring muscle weakness. Many of these tests have not been validated and can lead to people following restricted diets for long periods, often unnecessarily. The most reliable way of determining food intolerance is to withdraw a food from the diet and see if there is an improvement in symptoms.

Causes of food intolerance

There are several different causes of food intolerance as listed below.

Digestive enzymes Some people are sensitive to particular foods because they lack the right substances in the gut, called enzymes, to digest them. An example of this would be the lack of the digestive enzyme lactase, that is needed to break down the milk sugar lactose (see page 21).

Vasoactive amines These naturally occurring substances cause the blood vessels to narrow, which can lead to headaches, nausea, and giddiness. Foods rich in vasoactive amines include cheese, yeast extract, chocolate, red wine, and fermented foods.

Monosodium glutamate (MSG) This flavor enhancer is found in Chinese cooking and many processed foods. Large amounts of MSG can give headaches, flushing, abdominal discomfort, chest pain, and palpitations.

Irritants Some hot spices irritate the lining of the gut.

Gut bacteria There is growing evidence that the bacteria in our guts play a role in our health (see pages 36–7). Research suggests that the type of bacteria present in the large bowel may be linked with food intolerance.

SOME SYMPTOMS OF ALLERGY

- Swelling in the mouth and throat
- Runny nose (rhinitis)
- Watering eyes
- Breathing difficulties
- Skin rashes
- Small, itchy, red "nettle rash" (urticaria)
- Diarrhea
- Nausea and vomiting

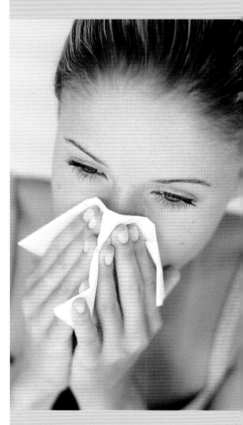

milk and dairy products

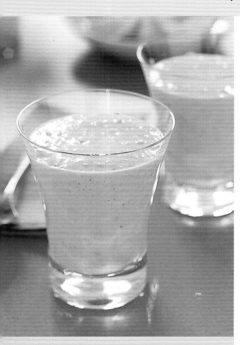

Milk is one of the most common foods linked to IBS. Research has found about 40 percent of IBS patients following an exclusion diet identified milk as the food that upset them. It is not clear why this is the case, but some people may have an intolerance to lactose (see page 21), which is the sugar found in milk.

Lactose

Lactose is made up of two sugars, glucose and galactose, and is broken down in the small intestine by an enzyme called lactase.

As infants we produce large amounts of lactase because milk is our main food. As we get older the production of lactase decreases. If there is not enough lactase to completely break down the lactose in the small intestine, it reaches the large intestine intact, where the gut bacteria ferment it. This can give rise to symptoms of diarrhea, bloating, pain, and wind.

Ethnic groups

People of Asian, African, and Mediterranean descent often have quite low lactase production, with 40–100 percent of the population affected. People from Scandinavia and northern Europe retain the ability to produce lactase, and the number of people with lactase deficiency in these areas is less, at around 5 percent.

"Lactase production is affected by a number of factors, including ethnicity, heredity, and previous illness."

Gastroenteritis

A bout of gastroenteritis can cause temporary damage to the lining of the small intestine and so upset the production of lactase. Some people find dairy products upset them after they have had a stomach upset.

lactose intolerance

The symptoms of lactose intolerance are very similar to those of IBS, and the number of people reported to have lactose intolerance and IBS ranges from 6 percent to 24 percent of the population. Research has shown that not everyone with a positive lactose breath test (see below) will improve on a low-lactose diet.

Many people with lactose intolerance can manage some lactose, sometimes as much as 1 cup milk a day, in their diet with no ill effects. A trial of a low-lactose diet for a couple of weeks may help people who include more than 1¼ cups of milk in their daily diet or if IBS symptoms started after a gut infection. In general, a milk-free diet gives better results than just excluding lactose.

Hard cheeses, such as cheddar, and butter have only a trace of lactose and can be included in a low-lactose diet.

Testing for lactose intolerance

There are several tests available to determine lactose intolerance, but the one most often used is called a lactose hydrogen breath test. A drink containing a known amount of lactose is taken after an overnight fast. Breath samples are collected before the patient takes the drink and then every 30 minutes afterward for two hours. If the lactose is not digested it will be fermented by the gut bacteria, which then produce hydrogen. The hydrogen enters the bloodstream and is eventually released from the lungs in the breath. A rise in hydrogen levels indicates lactose malabsorption.

MAIN SOURCES OF LACTOSE

- Milk (from a cow, goat, or sheep) and foods made with milk, such as custard, white sauce, milk puddings, yogurts, ice cream, and chocolate candy
- Lactose as a sweetener in foods and medications

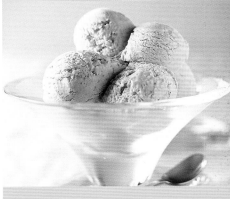

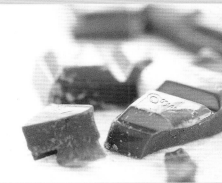

a milk-free diet

DIETARY SOURCES OF MILK

- Butter and margarine
- Cakes, cookies, and baked products
- Cheese
- Chips and savory snacks
- Chocolate
- Cream
- Ice cream, milk puddings, and desserts
- Pre-prepared meals and other convenience foods
- Vending machine drinks—hot chocolate, malted drinks, and milk shakes
- Yogurt

ALTERNATIVES TO MILK

- Cocoa, soy milk shakes, tea, coffee, fruit and herbal teas, fruit juices and cordials
- Milk-free cakes and cookies
- Milk-free margarine
- Plain nuts
- Ready-salted chips
- Rice milk (calcium enriched)
- Soy cheese and soy cream
- Soy milk
- Soy yogurts, soy desserts, and soy ice cream

Milk, whether from cows, sheep, or goats, is found in a wide range of foods—and often where you would least expect to find it. It is important to check food labels carefully to make sure that your food is milk free. This can be difficult because of the number of different words, all meaning milk, that can be used: milk proteins (casein, caseinates, lactalbumin, and whey), milk sugar (lactose), and milk fat (buttermilk). You should also keep an eye out for skim milk powder and milk solids.

Trial milk-free diet period

A trial of a strict milk-free diet for two or three weeks can help improve the symptoms of IBS, and keeping a food and symptoms diary (see page 31) is a helpful way of recording any changes in your symptoms. If there is no improvement after this time you should reintroduce milk to your diet.

Reintroduction of milk

If there is an improvement in the symptoms of IBS a gradual reintroduction of milk is recommended, starting with low-lactose dairy products, such as cheese or butter, and then moving on to milk itself, cream, and yogurt.

It is important to test one new food at a time and to have that food on two occasions during the day. Test the food for three or four days to allow enough time for any possible reaction to occur. If the symptoms return with the inclusion of milk it does not mean you will always have to avoid it. Many people find they can include small amounts of milk on an occasional basis with no problems. It is important to re-test foods after a couple of months as an intolerance to milk can be temporary and you might find you can manage it again.

Calcium intake

Milk and milk products are excellent sources of calcium, so it is essential to include alternative sources of calcium in the diet as well. This can be done by choosing other good dietary sources of calcium (see right). Calcium-enriched soy milk or rice milk are a good choice as they contain similar amounts of calcium to cow's milk. Aim to include two to three calcium-rich foods a day. Alternatively take a calcium supplement.

GOOD SOURCES OF CALCIUM

+ Baked beans

+ Breakfast cereals (some)

+ Broccoli, collard greens, watercress, and okra

+ Calcium-enriched soy and rice milks

+ Calcium-enriched soy cheese and soy yogurt

+ Canned sardines and pilchards (include the bones)

+ Sesame seeds and sesame paste (tahini)

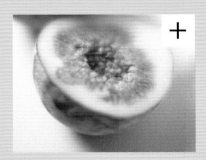

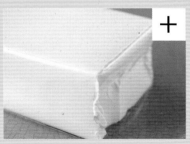

Meal plan for a milk-free diet*

Breakfast
■ Cereal with calcium-enriched soy milk with a tablespoon of dried fruit ■ Small glass of fruit juice

Lunch
■ Sandwich with milk-free margarine filled with meat or chicken or fish ■ Small mixed salad ■ Fruit or soy yogurt

Evening meal
■ Meat or chicken or fish or tofu ■ Vegetables or salad ■ Pasta, potatoes, or rice ■ Fruit salad with soy ice cream

Snacks
■ Fruit ■ Milk-free bun or cookie ■ Plain nuts ■ Ready-salted chips (occasionally)

* Remember to drink 6–8 cups of fluid every day.

wheat

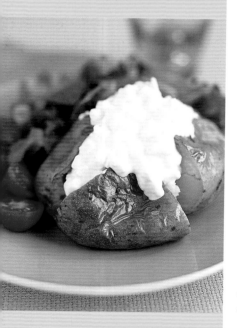

Wheat is another common food intolerance, and it has been identified by as many as 60 percent of people with IBS who have followed an exclusion diet. It is important not to confuse a wheat-free diet with a gluten-free diet.

Gluten versus wheat

Gluten is the name given to the protein found in wheat, rye, and barley. Oats contain a protein that is similar to gluten, and should initially be avoided if following a gluten-free diet. There is, however, some debate about whether complete avoidance of oats is necessary for everyone who needs a gluten-free diet. It is important to note that gluten-free foods are not always totally wheat-free as they often contain wheat starch. This makes them unsuitable for someone following a wheat-free diet.

Celiac disease

Celiac disease is caused by an allergy to gluten, which damages the lining of the small intestine. This can give rise to a range of symptoms, such as diarrhea, abdominal distension, pain, anemia, weight loss, fatigue, and recurrent mouth ulcers. Treatment is purely dietary through the long-term use of a gluten-free diet.

The symptoms of celiac disease and IBS are very similar, and it is important that celiac disease is ruled out before a diagnosis of IBS is given. While sensitive blood tests can indicate gluten sensitivity, they are not 100 percent accurate. The most reliable test is for a small piece of the lining of the small intestine to be removed by a doctor and looked at for signs of damage. Don't exclude gluten from the diet before these tests are carried out as this could give a negative result.

A wheat-free diet

A trial of a strict wheat-free diet can be helpful in IBS, especially if symptoms include abdominal bloating, diarrhea, and wind. Food labels can be confusing, and words that also mean "wheat" include wheat starch, bran, whole-wheat flour, flour, couscous, bulgar wheat, durum, semolina, spelt, and triticum.

Avoiding wheat for two or three weeks is an adequate length of time to see an improvement. Keeping a food and symptoms diary during this time will help confirm any changes (see page 31).

If there is no change in your symptoms it is unlikely that wheat is a problem, and it should be reintroduced to your diet. If there is an improvement you should reintroduce wheat to see if it causes problems again. Eat wheat twice during the day. Some people may experience symptoms within a day, but it can take up to a week for wheat to cause a reaction.

High-fiber wheat foods can cause abdominal bloating and wind, so try white bread and white pasta for three or four days before adding whole-wheat varieties.

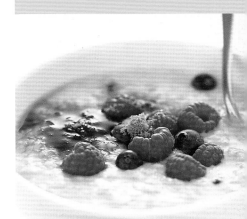

ALTERNATIVES TO WHEAT

The following list is not exhaustive, and you should always check the labels.

- Buckwheat pasta, corn pasta, and rice noodles
- Corn crackers
- Oatcakes
- Rice cakes
- Rye bread (100 percent rye flour)
- Rye crispbreads
- Wheat-free cakes and cookies
- Porridge, some granola, cornflakes, and rice crispies

Meal plan for a wheat-free diet *

Breakfast
- Porridge ■ Fruit smoothie

Lunch
- Baked potato with filling and salad ■ Yogurt or fruit

Evening meal
- Meat or chicken or fish ■ Vegetables or salad ■ Potatoes or rice or wheat-free pasta ■ Sorbet or fruit

Snacks
- Rice cakes ■ Oatcakes ■ Plain nuts ■ Fruit

* Remember to drink 6–8 cups of fluid every day.

exclusion diets

FOODS TO AVOID ON AN EXCLUSION DIET

- Beef, processed meats, pies, and pâtés
- Chocolate
- Citrus fruit and their juices and cordials
- Coffee, tea, cocoa, carbonated drinks, and alcohol
- Eggs
- Fish in batter or bread crumbs
- Milk (cow, goat, or sheep) products including yogurt, cheese, and ice cream
- Nuts
- Potatoes, onions, corn and vegetables canned in sauce
- Wheat, corn, rye, barley, and oats and all products made with them
- Yeast and yeast extract

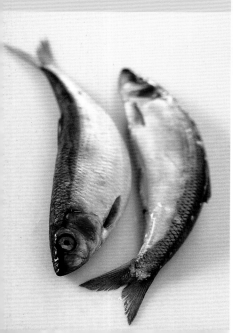

There is a group of people with IBS who find that they are intolerant of several different foods. These tend to be people who experience symptoms such as loose or frequent bowel motions, abdominal bloating, wind, and pain several times a week or even every day. Food intolerance is more likely in those people whose symptoms started after a severe bout of gastroenteritis or after having prolonged courses of antibiotics.

Adopting an exclusion diet

An exclusion diet excludes all the most commonly reported food intolerances in one go. It is a very restricted diet and should be followed with caution and preferably with the support of an experienced dietitian.

Typically, the basic diet is followed for two weeks, and it is essential that a food and symptoms diary is kept throughout this time (see page 31) to record if there has been any improvement over the exclusion period. If there is no change in symptoms over this time the diet should be stopped and a normal diet resumed. If there is an improvement then the excluded foods should be reintroduced back to the diet one at a time.

Are you prepared?

Although an exclusion diet can be helpful in identifying food intolerance it should not be undertaken lightly, as it can make life difficult.

Eating out can be tricky, especially during the initial two-week period. Don't be embarrassed to ask about ingredients used or if a meal can be adapted for you.

There are few ready-prepared foods available that are suitable for the basic diet, so be prepared to make meals from scratch—making them in bulk will save you time. Shopping may also take longer because you have to check food labels to make sure the product is free from all foods excluded on the basic diet.

Ensure your diet is nutritionally balanced by following healthy eating guidelines (pages 11–12) and by including a variety of foods on a daily basis. Take the opportunity to try new or unfamiliar foods and recipes.

Finding suitable snacks or eating away from home can be inconvenient or difficult, so you have to be organized and take suitable food with you.

FOODS ALLOWED ON AN EXCLUSION DIET

- All other meat, chicken, and game
- All other fruit, their juices and cordials
- All other vegetables, fresh, frozen, and canned
- Dairy-free margarine
- Fruit and herbal teas
- Rice milk (calcium-enriched)
- Rice, millet, quinoa, and buckwheat
- Seeds
- Soy milk (calcium-enriched), soy yogurts, soy ice cream, and soy cheese
- Sugar, syrup, and honey
- White and oily fish and shellfish

Meal plan for a basic exclusion diet *

Breakfast

- Rice cereal with sliced banana and calcium-enriched soy milk ■ Glass of apple juice

Lunch

- Cold chicken or ham with salad and rice cakes with dairy-free spread ■ Soy yogurt

Evening meal

- Pork chop with apple sauce ■ Vegetables and rice ■ Mixed berries with soy ice cream

Snacks

- Fruit ■ Seeds ■ Vegetable chips ■ Carob bar (check that it is milk-free) ■ Sesame snaps

Note The exclusion diet is not suitable during pregnancy or for women who are breastfeeding. If you are diabetic you should discuss the diet with your doctor before undertaking it.

* Remember to drink 6–8 cups of fluid every day.

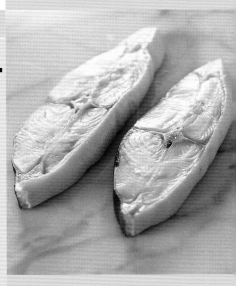

food reintroduction

"Pure foods need to be reintroduced before foods that contain them, such as yeast before wine and bread."

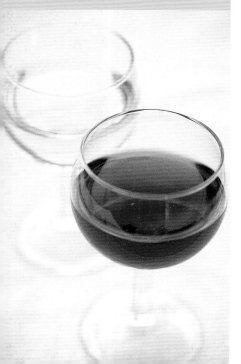

After two weeks on the exclusion diet food should be reintroduced to your diet. Take two days to test each food, as it can take 24–36 hours for a food to give a reaction. Wheat should be tested for seven days, because it can take longer for symptoms to return. If problems do occur, stop eating the food being tested and wait for symptoms to clear before trying the next food.

One food at a time

The amount of food tested is important. Having a small portion of a food once during the day may not be enough to give a reaction, so it is usually suggested that two portions of the test food are eaten. Also, don't test more than one food at a time, because this can lead to confusion and prolong the time on the exclusion diet.

Some test foods are found as ingredients in other foods, so it is important that these are tried first—for example, yeast needs to be tried before wine or bread and milk before cheese, yogurt, or butter.

Once the food reintroduction phase is complete the foods that provoke symptoms should be avoided for another three to six months. After this time it is advisable to re-test these foods, because quite often people find they are able to tolerate them after they have been avoided for a long period.

It is unusual to find more than three or four foods that cause symptoms. However, sometimes many foods appear to cause problems. For this group of people an assessment by a dietitian is strongly recommended to make sure that their basic diet is nutritionally adequate and to give advice on suitable alternatives to the foods that are being avoided.

Suggested order of food reintroduction

Food	Suggested amount for one portion *
Potatoes	1 large baked potato; 2–3 egg-sized boiled potatoes; 2 serving spoons of mash (use milk-free margarine); a small portion of fries cooked in suitable oil; 2–3 egg-sized roast potatoes
Beef	3–3$\frac{1}{2}$ oz
Yeast	3 brewer's yeast tablets a day
Cows' milk	A minimum of 1$\frac{1}{4}$ cups during the day, preferably 2$\frac{1}{2}$ cups a day; can be tested as whole, lowfat, or nonfat milk; use it in drinks or as an ingredient in dishes such as rice pudding
Rye	3–4 rye crispbreads; 1–2 slices of rye bread if yeast is tolerated (check that it is 100 percent rye flour)
Tea	No more than 4–5 cups a day
Butter or margarine	2–4 tablespoons during the day
Corn	4 tablespoons of cornflakes; 2 tablespoons of corn kernels or 1 corn cob; cornstarch in sauces; 2–3 corn crackers; vegetable oil can also be included
Eggs	2 during the day; egg as an ingredient in other food
White wine	A maximum of 3 glasses a day if yeast is tolerated
Citrus fruits	1 orange; $\frac{1}{2}$ a grapefruit; small glass of citrus fruit juice; 2 satsumas, tangerines, mandarins, or clementines; lemon juice in cooking; citrus fruit concentrates
Oats	3–4 oatcakes; 3–4 tablespoons of rolled oats for porridge; 1 piece of flapjack
Chocolate	3–4 teaspoons of cocoa; 3–4 teaspoons of hot chocolate powder; 2 oz chocolate if milk tolerated
Cheese	1–1$\frac{1}{2}$ oz; cheese made with goats' or ewes' milk should be tested separately
Wheat	1–2 slices of bread (if yeast is tolerated); 5–6 tablespoons of pasta; 2 Weetabix or Shredded Wheat; 4 tablespoons bran flakes
Coffee	No more than 3–4 cups a day
Yogurt	1 small carton or 3 tablespoons; yogurt made with goats' or ewes' milk should be tested separately
Nuts	A small handful unsalted or salted nuts; choose the type you would most commonly eat
Barley	Pearl barley in a casserole; barley water concentrates; 3–4 tablespoons breakfast cereal containing barley
Vinegar	In salad dressing, sauces, or added to food
Carbonated drinks	No more than 3 glasses (2$\frac{1}{2}$ cups) a day

* You need to have two portions a day unless otherwise stated

other diet-related triggers

SOURCES OF SORBITOL

- Fruit: plums, cherries, pears, and prunes
- Diabetic products: marmalade, jelly, and chocolate
- Sugar-free products: chewing gum and mints

SOURCES OF FRUCTOSE

- Fruit, such as apples, bananas, cherries, grapes, and pears
- Dried fruit, such as apricots, currants, figs and raisins
- Fruit juices, such as apple, grape, grapefruit, and prune

TIPS FOR CUTTING FAT INTAKE INCLUDE

- Broil, bake, steam foods rather than fry them
- Change to low-fat products
- Trim visible fat from meat and take the skin off chicken
- Avoid pastry
- Steer clear of creamy sauces and try tomato-based ones instead
- Limit your intake of chips, savory snacks, chocolate, cookies, and cakes to a couple of times a week

Some evidence suggests that some people with IBS are sensitive to certain sugars found within foods, such as fruit sugar (fructose) and milk sugar (lactose) and a sugar-alcohol called sorbitol. Fatty foods can also cause IBS symptoms.

Sorbitol

Sorbitol, often used as a sweetener in sugar-free and diabetic products and some medications, is also found naturally in certain fruits. An intake of about 1 oz a day is known to give stomach cramps, flatulence, and diarrhea, but lower intakes can cause symptoms.

Fructose

Some people with IBS complain of abdominal bloating and discomfort after being given fructose under test conditions. There is, however, no evidence that this is due to a true malabsorption of fructose, but it is thought that some IBS sufferers may have a heightened sensitivity to it. If foods rich in both fructose and sorbitol are eaten symptoms may be seen with much smaller portions of food.

Fatty foods

Rich or fatty foods are often linked with bowel problems. When fat is eaten it causes the body to release a substance called cholecystokinin (CCK)—a stimulant of colonic motility. This can cause pain, which is often mistaken for gallstones. Fatty foods can also give indigestion, abdominal discomfort, and diarrhea.

Spicy foods

Highly spiced foods have also been linked with indigestion, abdominal discomfort, and diarrhea.

the symptom-linked approach

Unfortunately, there is no one treatment for the symptoms of IBS, and everyone responds differently to different treatments. However, identifying the main symptoms allows you to follow a more structured approach in finding the most appropriate way of controlling them. The use of a food, lifestyle, and symptoms diary can prove helpful in identifying any patterns between diet and symptoms, stress or a combination of factors. Women can also find it worth making a note of their menstrual cycles.

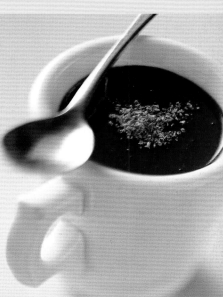

Keeping a symptoms diary

A small notebook is ideal for a symptoms diary, but some people prefer to keep it on their computer. You will need to keep the diary for a minimum of two weeks, although longer will be necessary if you experience symptoms less frequently than that or if there is a possible link to your menstrual cycle. You will need to keep a note of the information listed (see right).

Using the information

The information recorded in the diary will help you in a number of ways.

First of all, it will identify the main symptoms you are suffering and how often you are experiencing them. The diary should help you spot a link between a particular food and your symptoms, perhaps helping you identify if there is a link with fatty, spicy or rich foods, for example.

DIARY NOTES

- The time of eating, any symptoms, or any other event
- A general description of the food eaten at each meal—for example, white pasta with tomato sauce rather than just "pasta"
- The fluid taken—that is, the type of drink (including alcohol) and the amount
- A clear description of the symptoms—pain on right-hand side, loose bowel motion, hard, pellet-like motion, needed to rush to the toilet, and so on
- If you have had a particularly stressful or emotional day
- If you have taken any exercise or have been sitting down all day

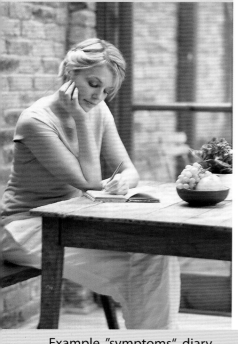

It will also reveal if you have an irregular meal pattern or if you eat differently during the week and highlight if you have a low- or high-fiber diet or if your intake of fiber alters a lot from day to day.

The diary will help you work out if you are having enough to drink and show if you are having too many soda drinks, caffeine, or alcohol. It will also make you think about the portion sizes of your meals and how you eat your food.

Noting how you feel will enable you to see if stress or anxiety play a part, and the diary will also reveal if the amount of exercise—or lack of exercise—has any effect on your symptoms.

Once you have established which are your main symptoms, you will be in a much better position to decide on the best way of changing your diet to help you manage your IBS.

Example "symptoms" diary

Date	Time	Food eaten	Time	Symptoms and comments
Mon 26	7.30 am	2 slices white toast with butter and jelly; cup of tea		
	During morning	3 cups of coffee and 1 apple	11.00 am	busy at work, feel stressed
		missed lunch		
			2.00 pm	headache, tummy pains
	3.00 pm	2 cups of tea and a candy bar		
	7.00 pm	chicken with new potatoes, peas, and broccoli; yogurt; glass of red wine		
	8.00 pm	glass of red wine		
	9.00 pm	cup of tea and a cookie		

symptom-linked groups

Although the symptoms of IBS vary from person to person, there are three main groups of symptoms into which most people fit. The three groups are: mostly diarrhea; episodes of diarrhea then constipation (alternating bowel habit); and mostly constipation. There may also be other symptoms present, such as abdominal pain or discomfort, abdominal bloating, flatulence, urgency to open the bowels, indigestion or acid reflux, tiredness, and headaches.

Before making any radical changes to your diet it is important that you are following a healthy, balanced diet with an adequate fluid intake (see pages 11–13). Don't forget the importance of regular meals, taking time over eating and moderating your portion sizes. Quite often symptoms improve just by making these simple changes. It is also important to allow time for your body to get used to any dietary changes. Improvements are unlikely to happen overnight, and it may take several weeks to notice a change. Continuing with a food and symptoms diary will be helpful because it will highlight if there has been any improvement in symptoms or not.

Mostly diarrhea

If you are in this group your main symptom is loose, frequent bowel motions at least once a week. Other symptoms may include abdominal bloating, abdominal discomfort or pain, flatulence (wind), and urgency to open the bowels.

DIETARY CHANGES FOR ALL SYMPTOM GROUPS

No matter which symptom group you are in, before you make any major changes to your diet it is important to:

- Follow a healthy, balanced diet
- Have an adequate fluid intake (6–8 cups of fluid a day)
- Have a regular meal pattern
- Keep a food and symptoms diary
- Check excessive intakes of caffeine, alcohol, spicy foods, fatty foods, fructose, and sorbitol

MAINLY DIARRHEA GROUP

- Low-fiber diet
- Single-food exclusion
- Exclusion diet

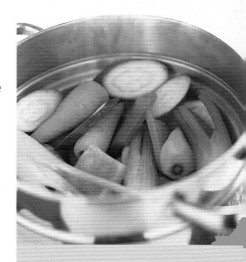

ALTERNATING DIARRHEA AND CONSTIPATION GROUP

Alternating bowel habit without wind and bloating

- High-fiber diet with the addition of a bulking agent if needed
- Single-food exclusion
- Exclusion diet

Alternating bowel habit with wind and bloating

- Low-fiber diet with bulking agent if needed
- Single-food exclusion
- Exclusion diet

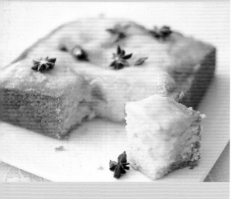

The first dietary change to make is to follow a lower-fiber diet (see pages 15–17) for three or four weeks. The addition of a fiber supplement or a bulking agent (see pages 15–17) may be necessary to prevent constipation. If there is no improvement after four weeks it is important to return to a normal diet.

If a low-fiber diet is unsuccessful it might be that a particular food is causing your symptoms. This is more likely if IBS started after gastroenteritis or a stomach upset, or after a long course of antibiotics, and diarrhea is occurring several times a week. Reviewing your symptoms diary may give you an indication of which food is responsible. The most common intolerances are milk and wheat, and a trial of a milk-free or a wheat-free diet—or both—can prove helpful (see pages 22–5). If your symptoms occur every day a full exclusion diet (see pages 26–7) might be the best approach.

Alternating diarrhea and constipation

If you are in this group your main symptom is loose or frequent bowel motions, followed by several days or weeks of a normal regular bowel habit. You will then find your bowel motions become less frequent and the motions become hard and pellet-like and more difficult to pass. Other symptoms may include abdominal bloating and flatulence (wind).

If you switch from diarrhea to constipation with no abdominal bloating and wind, try to gradually increase your fiber intake. At the same time make sure that you have an adequate fluid intake (see page 13).

If you find increasing your dietary fiber difficult the use of a fiber substitute or bulking agent (see pages 15–17) can be helpful. It is important to follow a high-fiber diet for several weeks and to keep a food and symptoms diary to monitor any change in symptoms. If increasing fiber intake is not helpful after about four weeks try an exclusion diet (see pages 26–7).

For those people who have an alternating bowel habit accompanied by abdominal bloating and wind a lower-fiber diet is often helpful (see pages 15–17). Again, a good fluid intake is essential. To prevent constipation becoming worse a bulking agent will help regulate bowel motions until higher-fiber foods are reintroduced to the diet (see pages 16–17). If there is no improvement after four weeks it is possible that there is a food intolerance and trying a single-food exclusion or a full exclusion diet can prove helpful.

Mostly constipation

The main symptom of people in this group is an infrequent bowel motion that can be painful to pass. Other symptoms may include abdominal bloating, abdominal pain, and flatulence (wind).

One person may say they are constipated if they don't pass a bowel motion every day, whereas another may say they are constipated if they open their bowels once a week. Generally, it is described as a bowel motion less than twice a week with the passage of hard, pellet-like or thin, flat, ribbon-like motions. Straining to pass a stool is often experienced together with abdominal pain.

Some people have sluggish bowels and need regular laxatives to stimulate a bowel motion. Such people should be under the supervision of a doctor. The continued use of laxatives is not recommended as the body can become dependent on them, and increased amounts are needed to have the same effect.

Where constipation without bloating and wind is the main symptom it is important to have an adequate fiber and fluid intake (see pages 13 and 15).

If constipation is the main symptom with abdominal bloating and wind, a lower-fiber diet plus a daily bulking agent, such as psyllium husks or linseeds (see pages 15–17), can help to improve symptoms.

MAINLY CONSTIPATION

Constipation without bloating and wind

- High-fiber diet

Constipation with bloating and wind

- Low-fiber diet with bulking agent if needed

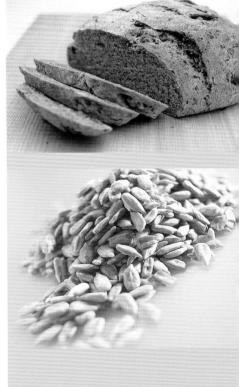

probiotics and prebiotics

GOOD SOURCES OF PREBIOTICS

+ Barley
+ Green vegetables
+ Jerusalem artichokes
+ Oats
+ Whole grains

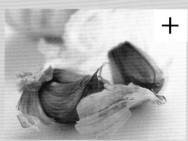

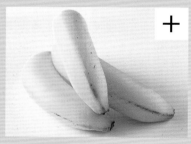

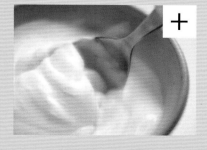

Everyone has billions of bacteria living in their large bowel. There are hundreds of different types of bacteria that in general live in a balance together. Certain types of bacteria—"good" or "friendly" bacteria—are beneficial to the body. They also help to keep harmful bacteria under control.

Upsetting the balance

When the balance of good and bad bacteria is altered it can lead to problems such as diarrhea, bloating, wind, constipation, discomfort, and generally feeling below par. This balance can be altered if you take antibiotics, or after a bout of food poisoning or "traveler's" diarrhea. It can also be affected by a diet that contains little fruit and vegetables but is high in fat and alcohol.

What is a probiotic?

Probiotic is the name given to live "good" bacteria. These can be taken as a supplement or added to food items. They are available in a wide range of products, including yogurts and yogurt drinks, and they are added to fruit juices and are available in capsule form. There is a lot of interest in the use of probiotics, and there is growing evidence that they:

☐ Boost the immune system
☐ Increase resistance to infection
☐ Help in the prevention and treatment of diarrhea resulting from bacterial infection
☐ Help to prevent diarrhea resulting from antibiotic therapy
☐ Improve movement of the bowel
☐ May improve mild inflammation of the bowel

At present there are no guidelines on the amount of probiotic that should be taken. More research is needed to work out how much and which types of bacteria are needed and the best way that they can reach the large intestine unharmed.

What is a prebiotic?

A prebiotic is a food substance that specifically promotes the growth of good bacteria in the bowel. These foods need to resist being digested in the small intestine so that they arrive relatively unchanged in the large bowel. The most commonly used ones are fructo-oligosaccharides (FOS) and inulin. Many probiotic supplements or foods now have prebiotics added to them as well.

Who needs probiotics and prebiotics?

Research shows that probiotics are a promising therapy for a wide range of health problems, including IBS, lactose intolerance, and gastrointestinal infections. Probiotics may also lower cholesterol levels and reduce the risk of cancer.

A trial of a probiotic may be worth undertaking if you have recently had an upset stomach or have started a course of antibiotics that has triggered your IBS. In general, they are safe to take for most people of all ages. However, if your immune system is not working properly or if you are taking drugs that affect your immune system—some cancer treatments, for example—you should avoid probiotics.

Capsules that have a combination of probiotics and a prebiotic, which have a special coating that resists digestion in the stomach, are a good choice. Yogurts and yogurt drinks must be kept chilled, and the longer they are kept the more likely it is that the bacteria will die. These yogurts are not suitable for people with a milk intolerance.

A GOOD PROBIOTIC WILL NEED TO:

- Contain bacteria that can reach the large intestine without being damaged
- Contain large numbers of bacteria
- Be taken on a daily basis
- Have more than one type of bacteria, such as *Acidophillus* and *Bifidobacteria* bacteria

some questions answered

Is there any drug treatment for IBS?
▶

There are various types of medication available to help control the symptoms of IBS; however, they do not cure the problem. These include:

- ☐ Anti-spasmodics to decrease muscular spasm in the gut
- ☐ Laxatives to treat constipation
- ☐ Medications to slow down the movement of the gut to control diarrhea
- ☐ Pain relief to control abdominal pain and discomfort
- ☐ Tranquilizers, which appear to help improve IBS symptoms

Most medications have unwanted side-effects, and not all medications are suitable for all people. You should discuss possible drug treatments with your doctor or pharmacist to ensure it is right for you.

Will I always have IBS?
▶

Most people find that their IBS symptoms come and go and that the symptoms become less severe with time. Symptoms are often triggered by a period of illness, stress, or upheaval.

It is important not to link all bowel symptoms with IBS. If you have a change in your symptoms, have rectal bleeding or blood in your stools, experience sudden unexplained weight loss, or a change to your normal bowel habit, you should have this checked by your doctor. These can be signs of more serious problems.

What is candida and is there a link with IBS?
▶

Candida albicans is a yeast-like fungus, which occurs naturally in the body. If the normal levels of bacteria in the gut are altered—which can happen after an infection or taking antibiotics—the candida can grow rapidly, resulting in thrush. Some people think this can lead to intolerance of yeast and yeast products and that avoiding them and sugary foods, which stimulate their growth, will improve symptoms of abdominal bloating, wind, and pain. There is, however, currently inadequate evidence to support the use of anti-candida diets in the management of IBS.

Do I need to take any vitamin or mineral supplements?
▶

If you follow a balanced diet it is unlikely that you will require any vitamin and mineral supplements. However, there are some instances when a particular vitamin or mineral may be needed, including:

☐ Calcium for people following a milk-free diet
☐ Multivitamin and mineral for those on an exclusion diet
☐ Iron, folic acid, or vitamin B12 for those who are anemic
☐ Evening primrose oil for those whose IBS symptoms are linked with their menstrual cycle

Multivitamin and mineral tablets often contain lactose (milk sugar), wheat, corn (maize), yeast, and other food items, so it is important that you choose a make that is suitable for your particular food intolerance.

Large doses of single vitamins and minerals are not recommended. Keep to ones that supply no more than the Recommended Daily Intake (RDI) unless otherwise advised by a doctor or dietitian. Excessive intake of certain vitamins and minerals can be dangerous or lead to unpleasant side-effects. For example, vitamin C in levels over 1 g can result in abdominal discomfort and diarrhea.

Does stress affect IBS?
▶

Yes, some people find that stressful situations can lead to diarrhea and abdominal pain. It can also lead to anxiety and a faster, shallow breathing pattern. Continued stress can give disturbed sleep and eating patterns, which in turn make IBS symptoms worse.

Finding a way to tackle stress, such as learning relaxation techniques and yoga, will help to decrease stress. Thirty minutes of moderate exercise five days a week is also helpful as exercise stimulates the body to produce feel-good substances called endorphins.

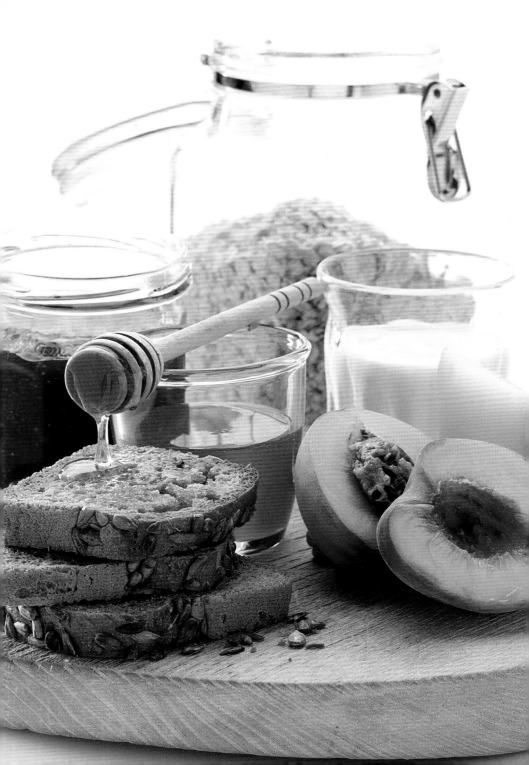

breakfasts

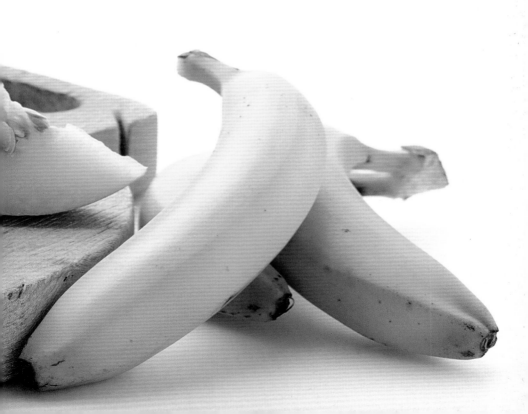

Nutrition
Gluten free, wheat free
Kcals 298
Fat 13 g
Saturated fat 6 g
Sodium 320 mg
Fiber 4 g

Preparation time
15 minutes
Cooking time
8–10 minutes
Serves
4

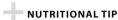 **NUTRITIONAL TIP**
Use stewed sliced peaches, nectarines,
or apples to lower the fiber content.

american cinnamon pancakes

Avoiding wheat and foods that contain gluten can limit breakfasts somewhat.
Topped with plain yogurt, mixed berries, and a drizzle of maple syrup, these thick,
griddle-style pancakes are lovely for a relaxed weekend breakfast.

1½ **cups frozen mixed berries**

2 **tablespoons water**

¼ **cup fine cornmeal (masa harina)**

¼ **cup tapioca flour**

½ **teaspoon ground cinnamon**

1 **teaspoon baking soda**

¾ **cup lowfat yogurt**

1 **egg**

1 **tablespoon sunflower oil**

Greek or whole milk yogurt, to serve

maple syrup or honey, to serve

1 Put the frozen fruit into a small saucepan with the measured water, cover and simmer for 4–5 minutes until hot.

2 Put the flours, cinnamon, and baking soda into a small bowl and stir together. Add the lowfat yogurt and egg and beat together briefly until just mixed and smooth.

3 Lightly oil and heat a large, nonstick skillet or griddle. Drop 6 large spoonfuls of the batter into the pan, spacing them well apart, and cook for about 2 minutes until the top has bubbled and the underside is browned. Turn it over and cook the other side in the same way.

4 Remove the pancakes from the pan, keep hot on a plate, add more oil if necessary and make 6 more pancakes in the same way. Serve 3 pancakes per portion, each topped with spoonfuls of fruit, some yogurt, and a drizzle of maple syrup or honey.

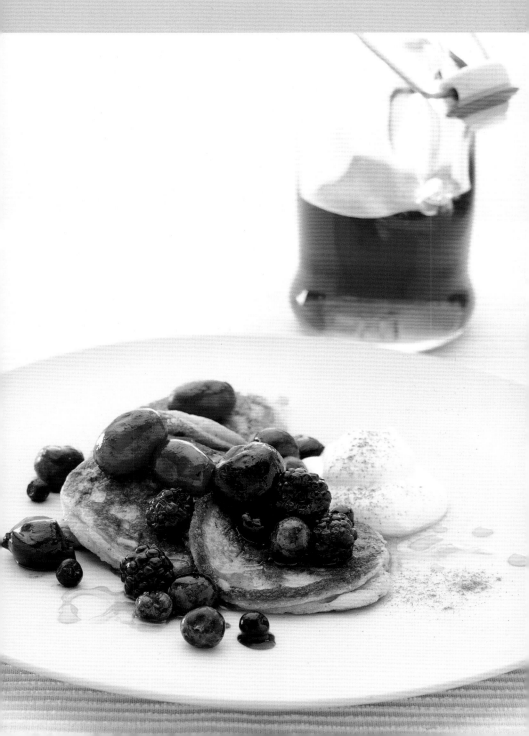

Nutrition

Wheat free, gluten free, high fiber

Kcals 343

Fat 8 g

Saturated fat 4 g

Sodium 127 mg

Fiber 5 g

Preparation time

5 minutes

Cooking time

4–5 minutes

Serves

4

NUTRITIONAL TIP

Use unsweetened soy milk instead of dairy milk if you prefer. If you use soy yogurt this dish will be suitable for an exclusion diet.

mixed grain porridge

Quick and easy to make, this blend of buckwheat, quinoa, and millet flakes gives a finished porridge that has a slightly smoother texture than one made from rolled oats.

½ **cup buckwheat flakes**

⅓ **cup quinoa flakes**

⅓ **cup millet flakes**

2½ **cups lowfat milk**

1¼ **cups water**

2 **bananas**

4 **tablespoons Greek or whole milk yogurt**

honey or maple syrup, to serve

sprinkling of ground cinnamon, to serve

1 Put the grain flakes, milk, and water into a saucepan and bring to a boil, reduce the heat and cook for 4–5 minutes, stirring until thickened.

2 Mash one of the bananas and slice the other. Stir the mashed banana into the porridge, spoon into bowls and top with spoonfuls of yogurt, the sliced banana, a drizzle of honey or maple syrup, and a sprinkling of cinnamon.

Nutrition

Dairy free

Kcals 229

Fat 6 g

Saturated fat 1 g

Sodium 120 mg

Fiber 3 g

Preparation time

15 minutes

Cooking time

15–20 minutes

Makes

10 muffins

✚ NUTRITIONAL TIP

Mixing whole-wheat and white flour is a good way to get the best of both worlds, but all whole-wheat or all white flour will work just as well—the fiber content either increases or reduces.

carrot and cinnamon muffins

Serve these muffins straight from the oven either plain or spread with a little lowfat cream cheese and apricot jelly for a special weekend breakfast treat. Any leftovers can be packed into lunchboxes or frozen for another day.

1 cup self-rising whole-wheat flour

1 cup self-rising white flour

½ cup dark brown sugar

1 teaspoon ground cinnamon

2½ tablespoons ready-chopped crystallized ginger or 1 piece stem ginger, drained and chopped

1¼ cups grated carrots

⅓ cup raisins or golden raisins

2 eggs

4 tablespoons sunflower oil

grated zest of 1 orange

6 tablespoons orange juice

3 tablespoons corn syrup

2 tablespoons barley flakes or rolled oats (optional)

1 Put the flours, sugar, cinnamon, ginger, carrots, and raisins into a mixing bowl.

2 Mix together the eggs, oil, orange zest and juice and add to the dry ingredients along with the corn syrup. Fork together until just mixed.

3 Line 10 sections of a deep muffin pan with paper bake cups and spoon the mixture into the cups. Sprinkle with barley flakes or oats (if used) and bake in a preheated oven, 375°F, for 15–20 minutes or until well risen and the tops are slightly cracked. Serve warm.

Nutrition

Dairy free, wheat free

Kcals 250

Fat 16 g

Saturated fat 2 g

Sodium 7 mg

Fiber 3 g

Preparation time

10 minutes

Cooking time

8–10 minutes

Serves

6

 NUTRITIONAL TIP

If you have a nut allergy, omit the nuts and add extra grains instead. If you omit the barley flakes and only use rolled oats, millet, and quinoa, this dish is suitable for an exclusion diet.

honeyed granola

This crunchy, caramelized breakfast cereal is packed with grains, nuts, and seeds. Serve it broken into pieces with dairy, rice, or soy milk or a mix of berry fruits and lowfat yogurt. Try adding a little ground cinnamon or ginger to the mixture before baking.

3 tablespoons honey

3 tablespoons sunflower oil

½ cup rolled oats or barley flakes

⅓ cup millet or quinoa flakes

½ cup mixed seeds, including 2 or more of sesame, sunflower, pumpkin, and flaxseeds

⅓ cup whole hazelnuts, cashew nuts, or almonds or a mixture, roughly chopped

1 Warm the honey and oil in a medium saucepan. Stir in the remaining ingredients and mix well.

2 Tip the mixture into a lightly oiled deep baking sheet or roasting pan and spread it into a thin, even layer. Roast in a preheated oven, 350°F, for 6–8 minutes.

3 Remove from the oven, stir well, moving the paler mixture from the center to the outer edges, and cook for 2 more minutes until evenly browned. Stir well.

4 Allow to cool, then transfer to an airtight storage jar. Keep for up to 7 days.

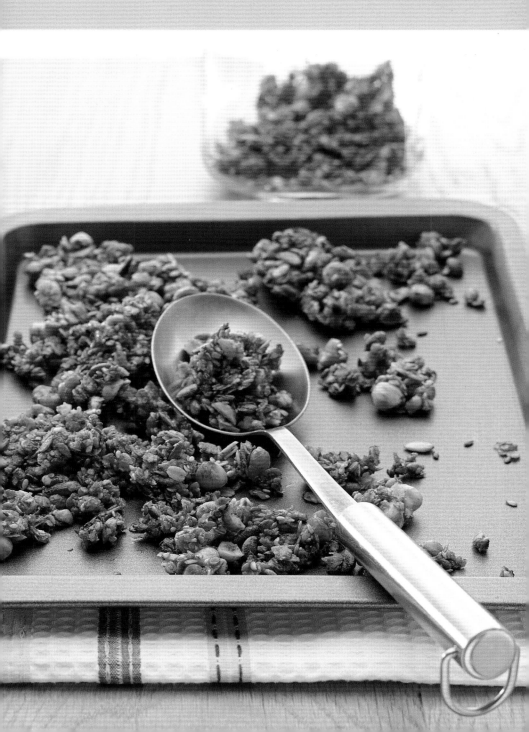

Nutrition
High fiber, milk free
Kcals 246
Fat 1 g
Saturated fat 0 g
Sodium 113 mg
Fiber 4 g

Preparation time
20 minutes, plus
soaking
Cooking time
about 1 hour 10 minutes
Makes
10 slices

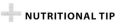 **NUTRITIONAL TIP**
This is a good choice for a low-fat, high-fiber snack or dessert.

pineapple, date, and golden raisin bread

This easy, yeast-free bread keeps well and is useful for those rushed mornings when you need a breakfast you can take with you. Serve thinly spread with butter or low-fat spread and have a banana or extra piece of fruit.

8 oz can pineapple slices in natural juice

12 pitted dates

1⅓ cups golden raisins

¾ cup pineapple juice

½ cup superfine sugar

1¼ cups self-rising whole-wheat flour

1¼ cups self-rising white flour

1 egg

1 Drain the pineapple and pour the juice into a small saucepan. Finely chop the pineapple slices and roughly chop the dates. Put the pineapple, dates, and golden raisins into a mixing bowl.

2 Add the measured pineapple juice to the juice from the can. Bring to a boil, pour over the fruit and allow to stand for 4 hours or longer if preferred.

3 Mix the remaining ingredients into the soaked fruit. Spoon into a lightly oiled and lined 6 cup loaf pan and level the top. Bake in a preheated oven, 325°F, for about 1 hour 10 minutes (check after 1 hour) or until well risen and a tester inserted into the center of the loaf comes out cleanly.

4 Allow to cool in the pan, then take out and peel away the lining paper. Wrap in foil or store in an airtight container for up to 7 days. Slice and serve plain or lightly buttered.

Nutrition

Dairy free, gluten free

Kcals 227

Fat 14 g

Saturated fat 3 g

Sodium 10 mg

Fiber 2 g

Preparation time

10 minutes

Cooking time

Serves

2

NUTRITIONAL TIP

Use soy milk and soy yogurt to make the drinks suitable for a milk-free diet.

minty avocado smoothie

If you are a reluctant fruit eater then one of these refreshing, vibrantly colored, vitamin-boosting drinks can be the perfect way to start the day.

1 ripe avocado, halved, pitted

3 stems of mint

juice of 1 lime

2 cups apple juice

1 Scoop the flesh out of the avocado skin into a blender or food processor. Add the mint, lime, and half the apple juice.

2 Blend until smooth and then add the remaining apple juice and mix briefly. Pour into 2 glasses.

ALTERNATIVES

Tropical sunrise Put into a blender or food processor 1 large ripe mango, pitted and peeled, 1 ripe nectarine or peach, quartered and pitted, 1¼ cups orange juice, and 1 tablespoon chopped crystallized or stem ginger. Blend until smooth. Pour into 2 glasses.

Spiced banana Put into a blender or food processor 1 large ripe banana, about 8 oz with skin on, thickly sliced, ¼ teaspoon ground cinnamon, 2 teaspoons honey, ½ cup plain yogurt and ¾ cup lowfat milk. Blend until smooth. Pour into 2 glasses.

Nutrition

Wheat and gluten free, low fiber

Kcals 187

Fat 8 g

Saturated fat 4 g

Sodium 197 mg

Fiber 1 g

Preparation time

15 minutes

Cooking time

30 minutes

Makes

10 slices

NUTRITIONAL TIP

If you don't need to avoid wheat or gluten, use white flour instead for a low-fiber treat.

quick cheese bread

Try this savory bread warm from the oven with sliced ham and tomatoes or toasted and cut into fingers with a soft-cooked egg for a tasty gluten-free breakfast. If you don't have any powdered mustard, mix 2 teaspoons Dijon mustard into the milk, but check that it is gluten free.

2 cups gluten- and wheat-free white bread flour with natural gum

¼ teaspoon salt

2½ teaspoons gluten-free baking powder

1 teaspoon gluten-free powdered mustard

1 cup grated mature cheddar cheese

1¼ cups lowfat milk

2 eggs

¼ cup reduced-fat spread, melted

1 tablespoon sesame seeds (optional)

1 Put all the dry ingredients into a mixing bowl and add the cheese. Put the milk, eggs, and melted spread into a large pitcher and fork together. Gradually mix into the dry ingredients and then stir until smooth.

2 Pour the mixture into a lightly oiled 6 cup loaf pan, level the surface and sprinkle with the sesame seeds (if used). Bake in a preheated oven, 350°F, for about 30 minutes or until well risen and a tester comes out cleanly when inserted into the center.

3 Allow to cool for 10 minutes, then loosen the edge of the bread and turn it out. Serve warm, cold, or toasted and spread with a little reduced-fat spread.

Nutrition

Wheat and gluten free, low fiber

Kcals 187

Fat 8 g

Saturated fat 4 g

Sodium 197 mg

Fiber 1 g

Preparation time

15 minutes

Cooking time

about 15 minutes

Serves

4

NUTRITIONAL TIP

If you are serving this dish to a vegetarian, omit the bacon and Worcestershire sauce, drizzling the mushrooms with a little balsamic vinegar instead. If you are on a gluten-free diet, you might want to omit the Worcestershire sauce, just in case.

brunch special

All the flavor of a fry-up but without the calories or fat, not to mention the indigestion afterwards. Choose deep, well-rounded mushrooms so that there is a good cavity to drop the egg into. If the mushrooms are quite flat put a large cookie cutter over the top of the mushroom or put the mushroom into an oiled individual tart pan so that the cutter or pan holds the egg in place.

4 deep field mushrooms, each a little over 3 oz

2 tablespoons reduced-fat spread

8 slices of Canadian bacon, 8 oz in total

4 tomatoes, halved

4 teaspoons Worcestershire sauce

4 eggs

salt and pepper

chopped chives, to garnish

multigrain toast (or white toast for a low-fiber diet), to serve

1 Remove the stems from the mushrooms and place the tops on a baking sheet, the black gills uppermost. Add a knob of spread to each and season. Lay the bacon over the top and arrange the tomatoes around the mushrooms.

2 Bake in a preheated oven, 400°F, for 10 minutes, then lift the bacon off the mushrooms and put it onto the baking sheet. Drizzle the Worcestershire sauce into each mushroom and break an egg in the center of each. Season the eggs, then return the baking sheet to the oven.

3 Bake for 4–5 minutes or until the eggs are just set and the bacon is cooked. Transfer to serving plates and sprinkle with chopped chives. Serve with multigrain toast.

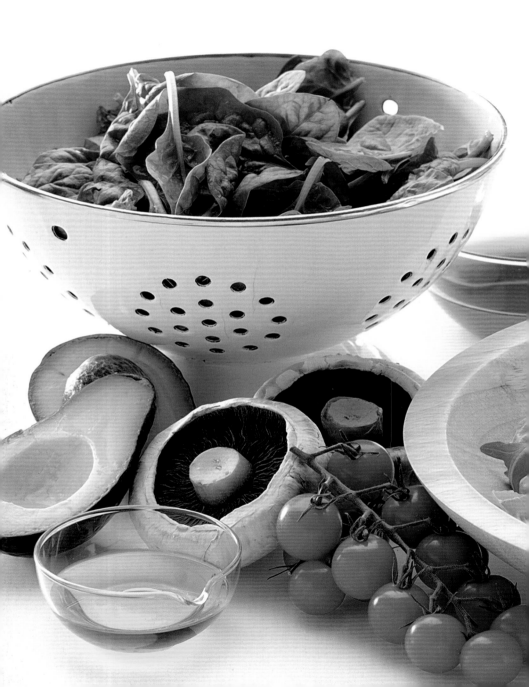

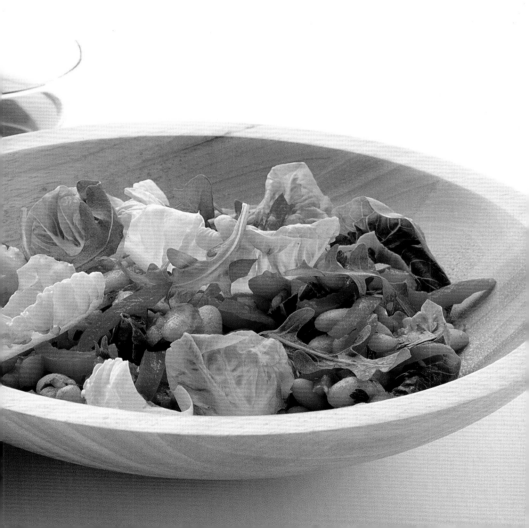

light
bites

Nutrition
Wheat and gluten free, high fiber
Kcals 270
Fat 13 g (2 g fat per 100 g)
Saturated fat 2 g
Sodium 210 mg
Fiber 5 g

Preparation time
25 minutes
Cooking time
about 40 minutes
Serves
4

✚ **NUTRITIONAL TIP**
If you are on a dairy-free diet, stir in
1¼ cups extra stock instead of the milk.
If eating wheat makes your symptoms
worse, make sure you use wheat-free
bouillon cubes or make your own stock
with a chicken carcass.

carrot and chickpea soup

Quick and easy to make, this soup uses ingredients that you will probably already
have in your pantry.

1 tablespoon sunflower oil

1 large onion, chopped

2½ cups diced carrots

1 teaspoon ground cumin

1 teaspoon fennel seeds,
roughly crushed

¾ inch ginger root, finely
chopped

1 garlic clove, finely chopped

13¼ oz can chickpeas, drained

5 cups gluten- and wheat-free
vegetable stock

1¼ cups lowfat milk

salt and pepper

GARNISH
⅓ cup slivered almonds

pinch of cumin powder

pinch of paprika

warm bread, to serve (optional)

1 Heat the oil in a medium saucepan, add the onion and fry
gently, stirring, for 5 minutes or until lightly browned. Mix in
the carrots, ground spices, ginger, and garlic and cook for
1 minute.

2 Mix in the chickpeas, stock, and a little salt and pepper,
bring to a boil, cover and simmer for 30 minutes or until the
vegetables are tender.

3 Puree the soup in batches in a blender or food processor
until smooth then return to the pan and stir in the milk.
Reheat gently.

4 Meanwhile, make the garnish. Heat the oil in a small
skillet, add the almonds, cumin, and paprika and cook for
2–3 minutes until golden-brown. Ladle the soup into bowls
and top with the almonds, cumin powder, and paprika. Serve
with warm bread, if desired.

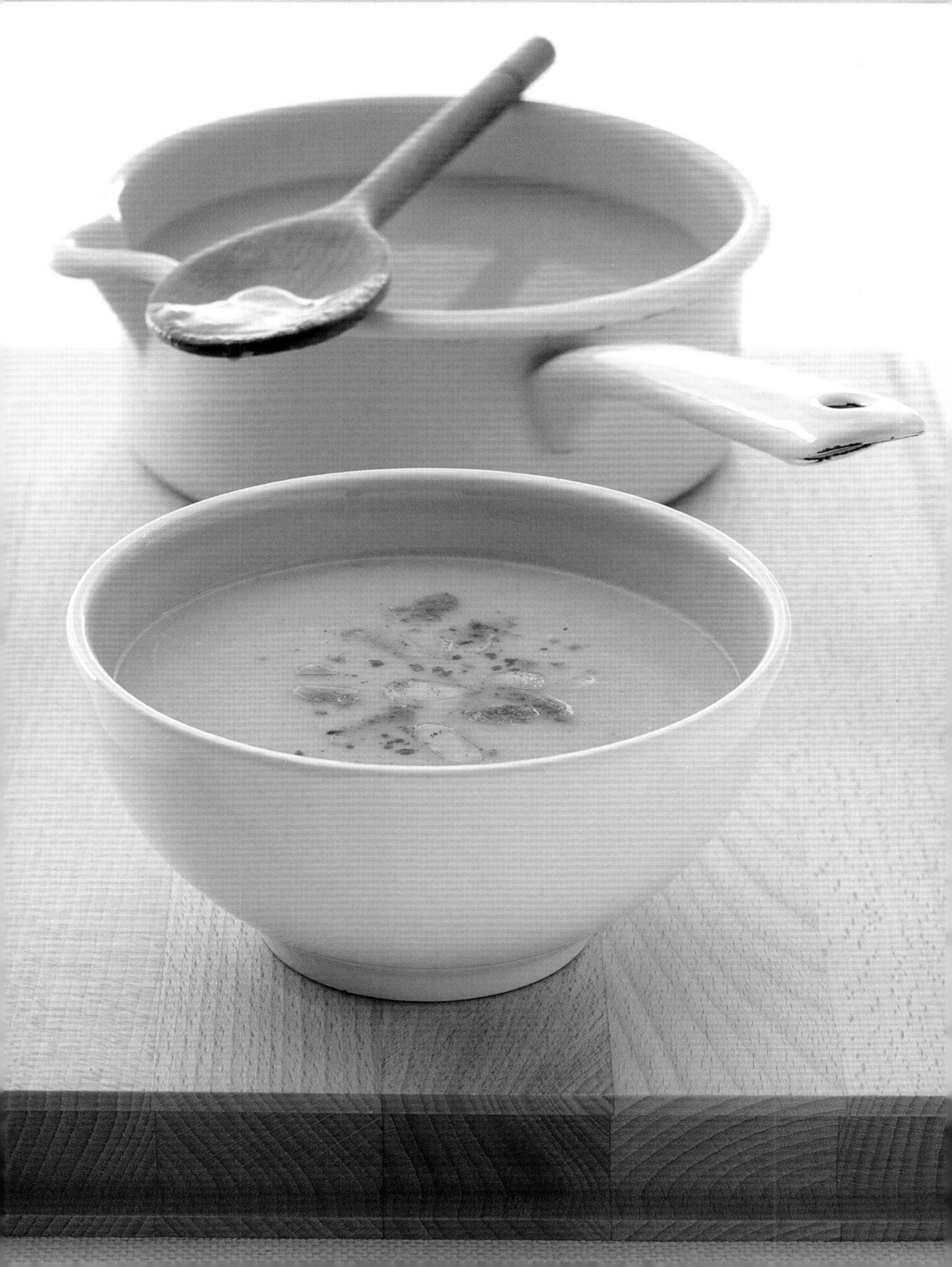

Nutrition
Wheat and gluten free, high fiber
Kcals 188
Fat 10 g
Saturated fat 4 g
Sodium 270 mg
Fiber 6 g

Preparation time
15 minutes
Cooking time
20 minutes
Serves
6

NUTRITIONAL TIP
Peas are a good source of soluble fiber.
If you are serving this dish to vegetarians,
omit the bacon garnish.

green pea and cilantro soup

Many people have a pack of frozen peas in the freezer, but how often do we use them for anything but a side dish? This quick and easy lunch is flavored with cilantro, but if you have some in the garden you might like to use mint instead.

1 tablespoon olive oil

1 onion, chopped

**1 baking potato, about
7 oz, diced**

**4 cups gluten- and wheat-free
vegetable stock**

2½ cups frozen peas

**about ¼ cup fresh cilantro
leaves**

3 slices of Canadian bacon

**6 tablespoons lowfat plain
yogurt**

salt and pepper

1 Heat the oil in a heavy saucepan, add the onion and potato and fry gently, stirring, for 5 minutes or until softened but not browned.

2 Mix in the stock and a little seasoning. Bring to a boil, cover and simmer for 10 minutes. Add the peas and cook for 5 minutes until the vegetables are tender and the peas are still bright green.

3 Puree the soup in batches in a blender or food processor until smooth, then return to the pan. Finely chop three-quarters of the cilantro, stir into the soup and reheat.

4 Meanwhile, broil the bacon until crisp and then cut it into strips. Ladle the soup into bowls, add a spoonful of yogurt to the top of each, lightly swirl into the soup and sprinkle with the bacon and remaining cilantro leaves.

Nutrition

Gluten free, low fat

Kcals 39

Fat 1 g

Saturated fat 0 g

Sodium 465 mg

Fiber 2 g

Preparation time

10 minutes

Cooking time

9 minutes

Serves

4

NUTRITIONAL TIP

If you are not avoiding foods that contain wheat or gluten, you could use soy sauce instead of tamari sauce. If you are preparing this dish for vegetarians, check that the curry paste does not contain shrimp paste; also, omit the fish sauce and add a little lime juice instead.

asian vegetable broth

There's no need to fry any of the vegetables first: simply add them to the flavored stock and simmer for a few minutes. To make this more filling, you could add some finely diced cooked chicken breast or frozen shrimp, which should be thawed first.

4 cups gluten-free vegetable stock

1–2 teaspoons red Thai curry paste (to taste)

1 tablespoon tamari sauce

2 teaspoons fish sauce (nam pla)

5 scallions, thinly sliced

1 garlic clove, finely chopped

1 carrot, about 4 oz, thinly sliced

4 oz button mushrooms, thinly sliced

3 oz broccoli, cut into tiny florets, stems sliced

2 oz snow peas, sliced

small bunch of fresh cilantro, torn into pieces

1 Put the stock, curry paste, tamari sauce, and fish sauce into a saucepan. Add the white part of the scallions, the garlic, sliced carrots and mushrooms and slowly bring to a boil. Reduce the heat and simmer for 5 minutes, stirring occasionally.

2 Add the broccoli and simmer for 2 minutes. Mix in the remaining green sliced scallions, the snow peas, and cilantro leaves. Simmer for 2 minutes, then ladle the soup into bowls.

Nutrition
Low fat
Kcals 207
Fat 5 g
Saturated fat 1 g
Sodium 222 g
Fiber 3 g

Preparation time
10 minutes
Cooking time
10–12 minutes
Serves
4

 NUTRITIONAL TIP
To increase the fiber levels in this dish, spread the wraps with hummus instead of the cheese or spoon the filling into warmed whole-wheat pita breads.

roasted vegetable wraps

Many people find raw peppers rather indigestible, but broiling and then skinning them solves the problem. Here the peppers are lightly flavored with pesto, then wrapped with lowfat garlic and herb cheese and peppery arugula leaves for a tasty lunch.

1 red bell pepper, quartered, cored, and seeded

1 yellow or orange bell pepper, quartered, cored, and seeded

2 zucchini, about 10 oz in total, sliced

4 teaspoons olive oil

1 teaspoon pesto

salt and pepper

4 large plain tortilla wraps

4 oz lowfat soft garlic and herb cheese

1 cup arugula leaves

4 teaspoons balsamic vinegar

arugula salad, to garnish (optional)

1 Put the peppers on a foil-lined broiler pan, skin side up, and arrange the zucchini around them in a single layer. Mix together the oil, pesto, and a little salt and pepper and brush over the vegetables.

2 Cook under a preheated hot broiler for 10–12 minutes, turning until the zucchini are lightly browned on both sides and the pepper skins are charred. Wrap the foil around the vegetables and set aside for 10 minutes.

3 Peel away and discard the softened skins from the peppers. Cut the pepper quarters and zucchini slices into strips. Warm the wraps according to the directions on the package, then spread the cheese in a strip down the center of each wrap.

4 Top with the cooked vegetables, arrange the arugula leaves on the vegetables and drizzle with the vinegar. Roll up tightly, cut in half, and serve immediately or wrap in plastic wrap and eat later, with extra arugula salad, if desired.

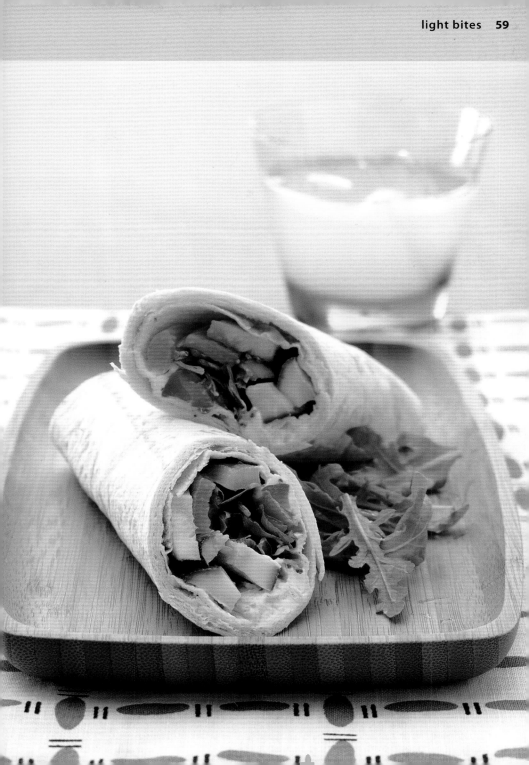

Nutrition
Wheat free, gluten free
Kcals 303
Fat 10 g
Saturated fat 3 g
Sodium 83 mg
Fiber 2 g

Preparation time
20 minutes
Cooking time
13–18 minutes
Serves
4

NUTRITIONAL TIP
Read the package carefully when you are
buying wasabi for the first time and make
sure that it is gluten free.

trout and new potato salad

Serve this salad while the potatoes and trout flakes are still warm; or, if you would
rather make it in advance, allow the potatoes and trout to cool and toss with the
dressing and salad leaves just before serving. Flaked smoked mackerel fillets
would taste good in this salad but avoid those coated in peppercorns or the salad
may be too fiery.

**1 lb baby new potatoes,
scrubbed, larger ones halved**

**1 lb trout fillets, rinsed and
drained**

²/₃ cup lowfat plain yogurt

**1–2 teaspoons gluten-free
wasabi (Japanese horseradish),
to taste**

2 teaspoons honey

salt and pepper

2³/₄ cups salad leaves

1 Half-fill the base of a steamer with water and bring to a
boil, add the potatoes to the water and put the fish fillets
in a single layer in the steamer above. Cover and cook for
8 minutes until the fish is just cooked and flakes easily
when pressed with a knife. Remove the top of the steamer,
re-cover the potatoes, cook for 5–10 minutes more or until
tender, then drain.

2 Transfer the fish to a plate or cutting board and break
it into flakes, discarding the skin and any bones.

3 Mix the yogurt with the wasabi, honey, and a little salt and
pepper in a salad bowl, add the warm potatoes and toss
together. Add the fish flakes and salad leaves and toss
together lightly. Serve immediately.

Nutrition

Dairy free, high fiber

Kcals 318

Fat 17 g

Saturated fat 2 g

Sodium 400 mg

Fiber 4 g

Preparation time

15 minutes

Cooking time

Serves

4

NUTRITIONAL TIP

Couscous is made from durum wheat, so, if you are avoiding wheat and foods that contain gluten, add cooked quinoa or millet grains instead.

couscous salad

Mix and match ingredients for this quick-to-put-together salad depending on what you have in the refrigerator. Canned or fresh salmon, diced cooked chicken, diced ham, or crumbled feta could also be added instead of the tuna.

1 cup couscous

2 cups boiling water

7 oz can tuna in spring water, drained

2 oz sun-dried tomatoes, drained and thinly sliced

¼ cup pitted black olives, roughly chopped

2 teaspoons capers, drained and roughly chopped (optional)

½ red onion, finely chopped

4 oz cherry tomatoes, halved

1 cup arugula or mixed salad leaves

DRESSING
3 tablespoons olive oil

juice of 1 lemon

small bunch of basil leaves, roughly torn

salt and pepper

1 Put the couscous in a bowl, pour over the boiling water and allow to soak for 5 minutes.

2 Flake the tuna into pieces and add them to the couscous with the sun-dried tomatoes, olives, and capers (if used). Add the onion and cherry tomatoes and fork together.

3 Mix together the ingredients for the dressing, drizzle over the salad and lightly toss together. Sprinkle the salad leaves on top and serve.

Nutrition
Wheat, gluten and dairy free
Kcals 500
Fat 25 g
Saturated fat 4 g
Sodium 913 mg
Fiber 4 g

Preparation time
20 minutes
Cooking time
8–10 minutes
Serves
4

 NUTRITIONAL TIP
Tamari sauce is the Japanese equivalent
of soy sauce and is wheat and gluten
free, but soy sauce can be used if you are
not avoiding wheat.

asian salmon salad

Packed lunches needn't mean just sandwiches. This tasty rice salad can be made the
night before and taken to work in an insulated lunch box. Use a large can of salmon
instead of freshly broiled salmon if you prefer, and snow peas or sliced green beans
can be used instead of the sugar snap peas.

³/₄ cup long-grain rice

4 salmon fillets, each
about 4 oz

3 tablespoons tamari sauce

4 oz sugar snap peas, halved
lengthwise

1 large carrot, cut into
matchstick strips

4 scallions, trimmed and thinly
sliced

1 cup bean sprouts, rinsed and
drained

6 teaspoons sunflower oil

3 tablespoons sesame seeds

2 teaspoons fish sauce
(nam pla) (optional)

2 teaspoons rice or white
wine vinegar

small bunch of fresh cilantro or
basil, torn into pieces

1 Half-fill a medium saucepan with water and bring to a boil.
Add the rice to the water and simmer for 8 minutes.

2 Meanwhile, put the salmon on a foil-lined broiler rack and
drizzle over 1 tablespoon of the tamari sauce. Cook under
a preheated broiler for 8–10 minutes, turning once, until
browned and the fish flakes easily.

3 Add the sugar snap peas to the rice and cook for 1 minute.
Drain, rinse with cold water and drain again. Tip into a salad
bowl and mix in the carrot, scallions, and bean sprouts.

4 Heat 1 teaspoon oil in a nonstick skillet, add the sesame
seeds and fry until just beginning to brown. Add
1 tablespoon of tamari sauce and quickly cover the pan so
that the seeds do not ping out. Take off the heat and allow
to stand for 1–2 minutes, then mix in the remaining tamari
sauce, oil, fish sauce (if used), and vinegar. Add the sesame
mixture to the salad and toss together. Take the skin off the
salmon and flake the flesh into pieces—discard any bones.
Add to the salad with the herb leaves. Serve warm or cold.

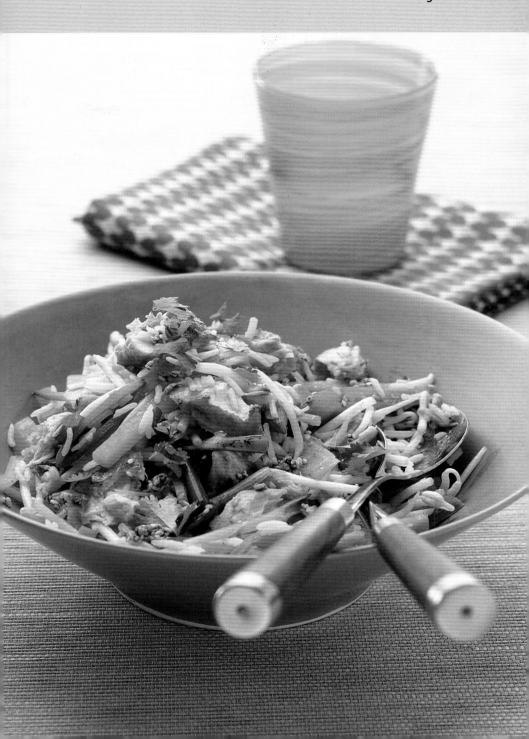

Nutrition
High fiber
Kcals 400
Fat 24 g
Saturated fat 7 g
Sodium 750 mg
Fiber 10 g

Preparation time
15 minutes
Cooking time
10–15 minutes
Serves
4

NUTRITIONAL TIP
Replace the feta cheese with tuna, salmon, or chicken to make a dish suitable for a dairy-free diet.

white bean, feta, and roasted pepper

This robust salad can be made in advance, so it's great for a healthy packed lunch. Take the salad leaves in a separate plastic bag to keep them crisp. The feta cheese could be omitted and a 6¼ oz can of drained and flaked tuna in spring water included instead.

2 red bell peppers, halved, cored, and seeded

4 tablespoons olive oil

2 tablespoons balsamic or red wine vinegar

3 teaspoons sun-dried tomato paste

4 teaspoons capers, chopped if large

salt and pepper

2 x 13¼ oz cans cannellini beans or navy beans or chickpeas, drained

½ red onion, finely chopped

4 sticks celery, sliced

4 oz feta cheese, drained

1 romaine lettuce

1 Put the peppers, skin side up, on a foil-lined broiler rack, brush with a little of the oil and cook under a preheated broiler for 10–15 minutes until the peppers are softened and the skins charred. Wrap in foil and allow to cool.

2 Meanwhile, make the dressing by mixing the remaining oil with the vinegar, tomato paste, capers, and salt and pepper.

3 Stir the drained beans or chickpeas, onion, and celery into the dressing. Peel the skins off the peppers then cut the flesh into strips. Add to beans and gently toss together. Crumble the feta cheese over the top and serve the salad scooped over lettuce leaves.

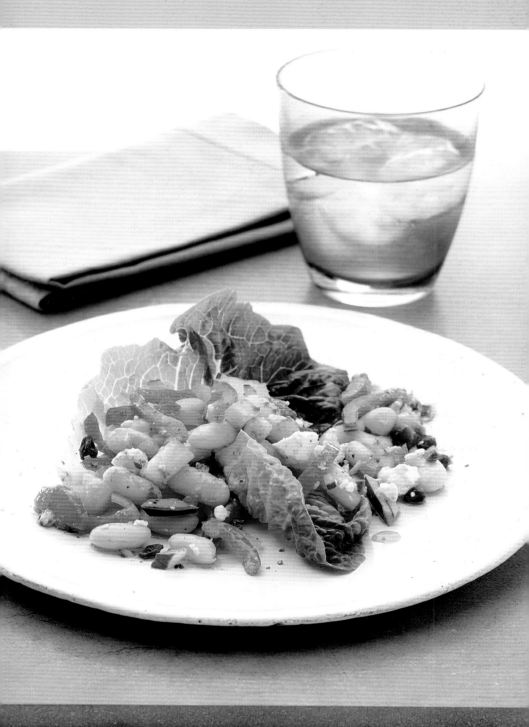

Nutrition
Gluten free, high fiber
Kcals 365
Fat 5 g (1 g fat per 100 g)
Saturated fat 3 g
Sodium 500 mg
Fiber 7 g

Preparation time
10 minutes
Cooking time
50–60 minutes
Serves
1

NUTRITIONAL TIP
These fillings taste just as good served with the traditional baked potato. If following a gluten-free diet, check that the sweet chili sauce and korma curry paste are gluten free.

sweet potato with cottage cheese and chili

We all love baked potatoes, but sweet potatoes make a lighter and more unusual lunch choice and, for those avoiding wheat and gluten, a tasty and filling alternative to sandwiches.

1 sweet potato, about 10 oz

½ cup cottage cheese

1 tablespoon sweet chili sauce

few fresh cilantro leaves

salt and pepper

1 Scrub and prick the sweet potato and cook it in a preheated oven, 400°F, for 50–60 minutes or until it is tender.

2 Cut the sweet potato in half then in half again to make a cross, fluff up the center with a fork, then top with cottage cheese, a little salt and pepper, a drizzle of chili sauce and some torn cilantro leaves.

ALTERNATIVES
Curried ham Mix together 3 tablespoons lowfat plain yogurt and 1 teaspoon korma curry paste in a small bowl. Stir in a little red onion, finely chopped, and a ¾ inch thick slice of cucumber, finely diced. Spoon over the top of 1 baked sweet potato (see above) and sprinkle with 1 large slice of ham, roughly diced.

Avocado salsa Mix together in a bowl ½ ripe avocado, pitted, peeled, and diced, the juice of ½ lime, a little red onion, finely chopped, ½ apple, cored and finely diced, 3 cherry tomatoes, quartered, and a few cilantro leaves, roughly chopped. Spoon the mixture over 1 baked sweet potato (see above).

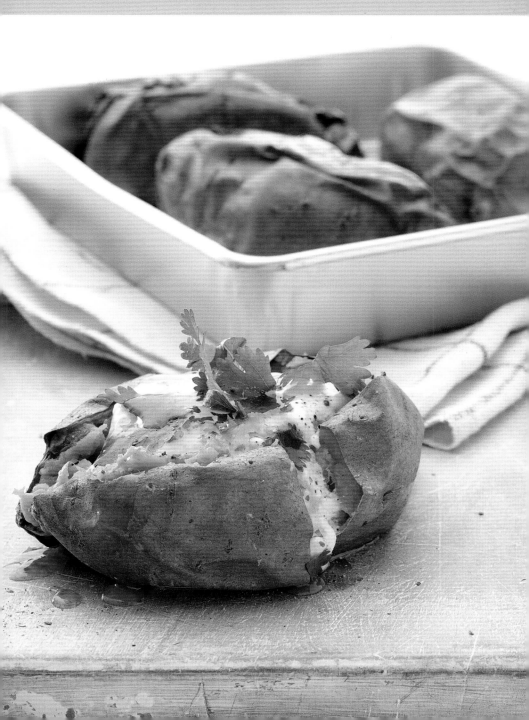

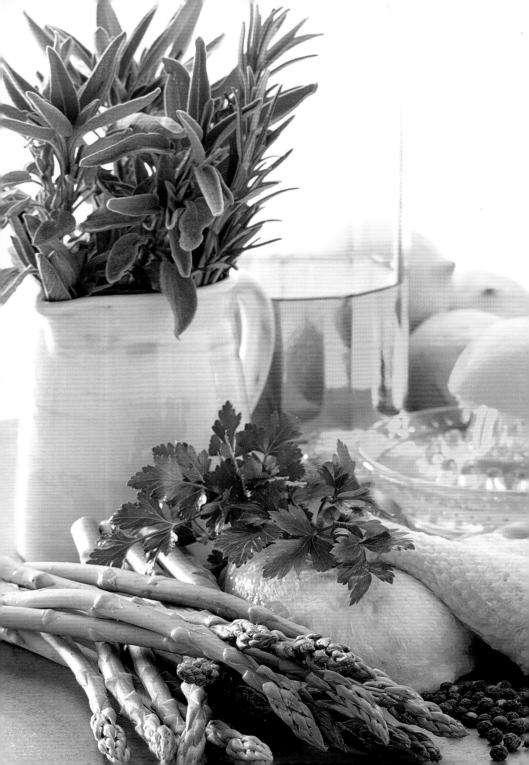

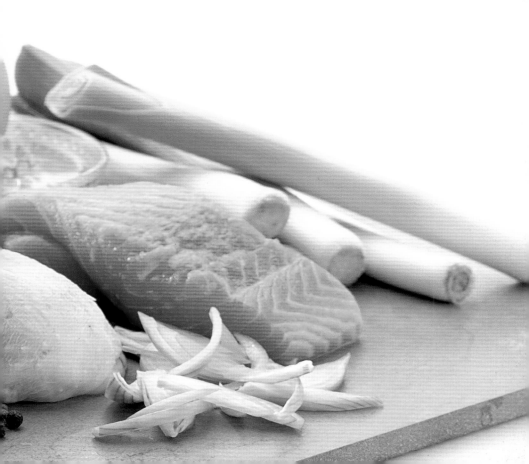

main
meals

Nutrition	Preparation time	NUTRITIONAL TIP
Low fiber	25 minutes	The salsa can be used with other dishes
Kcals 327	**Cooking time**	if you are on a milk- or wheat-free diet.
Fat 15 g	12–15 minutes	
Saturated fat 4 g	**Serves**	
Sodium 285 mg	4	
Fiber 2 g		

sticky chicken with salsa

Refreshingly fruity, this dish makes a lovely summer supper. Cook the chicken under the broiler or on the barbecue. The chicken can also be cut into cubes and threaded onto 8 skewers if you prefer. Use hot smoked Spanish pimento instead of paprika for a chili-like oomph.

4 boneless, skinless chicken breasts, about 1¼ lb in total

2 tablespoons tomato ketchup

1 tablespoon Worcestershire sauce

1 tablespoon sunflower oil

1 teaspoon Dijon mustard

1 teaspoon honey

½ teaspoon paprika

salt and pepper

green salad, to serve

new potatoes, to serve

SALSA
1 avocado, peeled and diced

1 small mango, peeled and diced

1 lime, grated zest and juice

2 tomatoes, skinned (if desired), seeded, and diced

½ small red onion, finely chopped

1 Rinse the chicken breasts with cold water, drain well, then put on a foil-lined broiler rack.

2 Mix together the tomato ketchup, Worcestershire sauce, oil, mustard, honey, paprika, and salt and pepper and brush over the chicken. Cook under a preheated broiler for 12–15 minutes, turning several times, until the meat is browned and cooked through.

3 Meanwhile, make the salsa. Mix the diced avocado and mango with the lime zest and juice, then stir in the tomatoes and onion.

4 Slice the chicken into strips and transfer to plates. Serve with spoonfuls of salsa, with a green salad and some baby new potatoes.

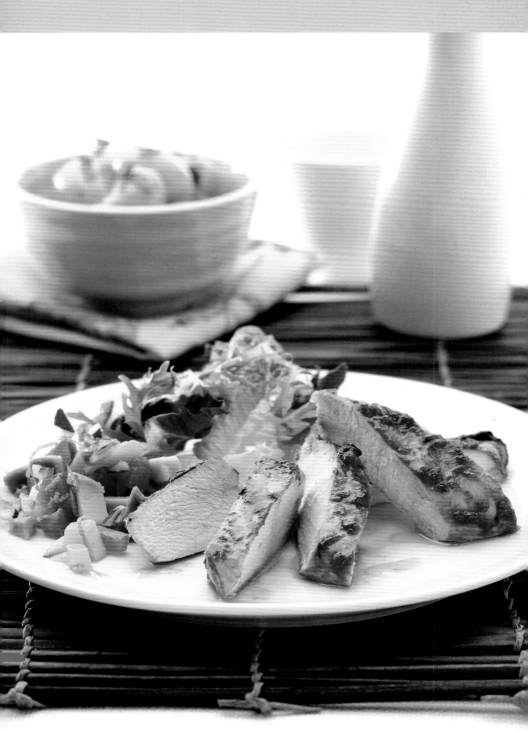

Nutrition

Dairy, wheat and gluten free

Kcals 372

Fat 13 g

Saturated fat 4 g

Sodium 636 mg

Fiber 9 g

Preparation time

20 minutes

Cooking time

about 2 hours

15 minutes

Serves

4

 NUTRITIONAL TIP

Either pepperoni or chorizo can be used in this recipe, but read the labels carefully if you are avoiding wheat products to make sure that they are definitely wheat free because some makes contain wheat.

slow-cooked chicken

This all-in-one supper dish is ideal for weekends. You can prepare everything, then pop the casserole in the oven, leaving you free to garden or play with the children without fear of it spoiling.

1 tablespoon olive oil

8 chicken thighs, about 2 lb in total, skinned, boned, and quartered

1 large onion, roughly chopped

1–2 garlic cloves, finely chopped

1 teaspoon hot smoked Spanish paprika (pimento)

13 oz can chopped tomatoes

2 cups wheat- and gluten-free chicken stock

13¼ oz can cranberry beans, drained

salt and pepper

2–3 stems of rosemary

1 lb baking potatoes, peeled, and diced

2 carrots, about 8 oz in total, sliced

3 oz pack sliced pepperoni

roughly chopped flat-leaf parsley, to garnish

1 Heat the oil in a large skillet, add the chicken a few pieces at a time, until all the pieces have been added, then cook over a high heat for 5 minutes until lightly browned. Drain and transfer to a casserole dish.

2 Add the onion to the pan and cook, stirring, for 5 minutes or until pale golden. Add the garlic and paprika and cook, stirring, for 1 minute. Mix in the tomatoes, stock, beans, rosemary, and salt and pepper and bring to a boil.

3 Add the potatoes, carrots, and sliced pepperoni to the casserole dish, then pour over the hot tomato sauce. Cover and bake in a preheated oven, 350°F, for 1½–2 hours until tender, adding a little extra stock if necessary. Spoon into bowls and serve sprinkled with parsley.

Nutritional value
Wheat free, gluten free
Kcals 560
Fat 24 g
Saturated fat 10 g
Sodium 235 mg
Fiber 4 g

Preparation time
20 minutes, plus
marinating
Cooking time
1 hour 40 minutes
Serves
4

NUTRITIONAL TIP
Cooking the potatoes in stock in a separate dish rather than roasting them around the meat makes a great low-fat alternative to roast potatoes. You will also need to strain any fat off the meat juices if you serve these with the dish.

yogurt-marinated roast lamb

Inspired by East European cooking, this unusual way of roasting a leg of lamb keeps it beautifully moist and full of flavor.

3–3¼ lb leg of lamb

2 garlic cloves, sliced

1 cup lowfat plain yogurt

1 tablespoon olive oil

4 teaspoons chopped dill

1 teaspoon caraway seeds

1 teaspoon mild paprika

1 teaspoon black peppercorns, roughly crushed

salt

1½ lb small baking potatoes, scrubbed

1 onion, sliced

7 cups hot wheat- and gluten-free lamb stock

1 tablespoon butter

1 Make slits at intervals over the lamb joint, cutting through the fat into the meat, and insert a slice of garlic into each slit. Transfer to a large non-metallic dish.

2 Mix together the yogurt, oil, dill, caraway, paprika, peppercorns, and salt and spread the mixture over the lamb. Marinate for 3–4 hours in the refrigerator.

3 Put the lamb on a roasting rack in a roasting pan. Thinly slice the potatoes and layer them in a shallow ovenproof dish with the onion and a little extra salt and pepper. Pour in 2½ cups hot stock. Dot the top with butter, cover with foil, and put on a high shelf in the oven.

4 Pour 2½ cups hot stock into the roasting pan and put the lamb under the potatoes in the oven. Roast in a preheated oven, 375°F, allowing 25 minutes per 1 lb plus 25 minutes. Check on the meat from time to time, and spoon stock over the lamb if it looks dry or cover with foil if it is browning too quickly. Top up the pan with extra stock as needed. Remove the foil from the potatoes for the last 30 minutes of the cooking time.

5 Transfer the lamb to a warmed serving plate, then strain the stock and meat juices from the pan into a pitcher. Serve with the baked potatoes.

Nutrition
Wheat and gluten free, high fiber
Kcals 420
Fat 26 g
Saturated fat 7 g
Sodium 180 mg
Fiber 6 g

Preparation time
10 minutes
Cooking time
8–10 minutes
Serves
4

 NUTRITIONAL TIP
Omit the lime juice and use soy yogurt
to make this dish suitable for a milk-free
or an exclusion diet.

seared salmon with garden greens

The summery green vegetables in this dish require the same cooking time, but you
could use broccoli, sugar snap peas, bok choy, spinach, or any other vegetable you like.
Make sure you put the vegetables that take the longest to cook in the steamer first.

**4 salmon steaks, each about
5 oz, rinsed and dried**

1 tablespoon olive oil

grated zest and juice of 1 lime

1 teaspoon honey

salt and pepper

**8 oz runner beans or green
beans, stringed, cut into
thin slices**

**8 oz bunch of asparagus,
trimmed, cut into
2 inch lengths**

1¼ cups frozen peas

6 tablespoons plain yogurt

4 teaspoons chopped mint

1 Put the salmon on a foil-lined broiler rack. Mix together the
oil, lime juice, honey, and salt and pepper and spoon over
both sides of the salmon. Broil the salmon under a preheated
broiler for 8–10 minutes, turning once, until it is browned on
both sides and the fish flakes easily into even-colored flakes
when pressed with a knife.

2 Meanwhile, steam the beans, asparagus, and frozen peas
for 5 minutes. Mix the yogurt with the chopped mint, lime
zest and a little salt and pepper.

3 Toss the just-cooked vegetables with the minted yogurt,
spoon into the center of 4 serving plates and arrange the
salmon on top. Garnish with extra small mint leaves, if
desired. Serve with new potatoes or rice.

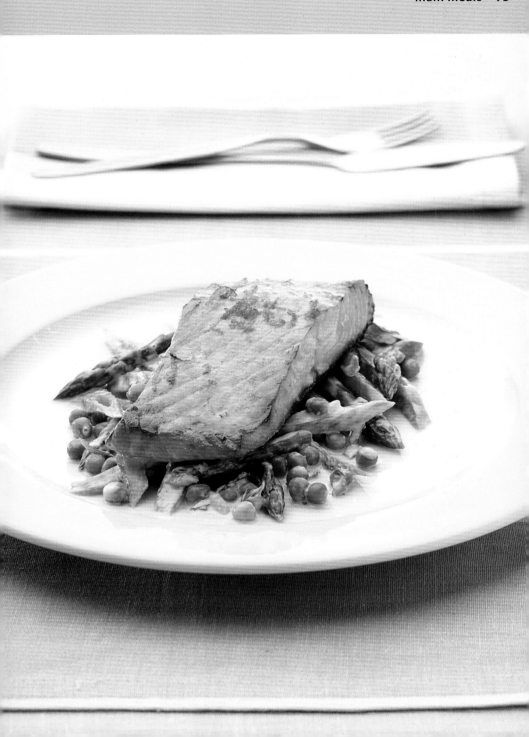

Nutrition
Wheat, gluten and dairy free
Kcals 593
Fat 31 g
Saturated fat 7 g
Sodium 1200 mg
Fiber 3 g

Preparation time
15 minutes
Cooking time
25–30 minutes
Serves
4

NUTRITIONAL TIP
Use white rice to make this dish suitable
for a low-fiber diet.

mixed fish kedgeree

If you have trouble persuading your family to adopt a healthier diet, this is a
good recipe to slip in. Because the brown rice is lightly spiced, they won't even
realize it is different.

1 onion, chopped

**2½ cups wheat- and gluten-
free fish or chicken stock**

1 cup easy-cook brown rice

½ teaspoon ground turmeric

**5 cardamom pods, roughly
crushed**

salt and pepper

10 oz smoked haddock

**10 oz package peppered or
plain smoked mackerel fillets**

**4 eggs, hard-cooked, shelled,
and quartered**

small bunch of fresh cilantro

1 Put the onion, stock, rice, turmeric, and cardamom pods
and the black seeds into a skillet with a little salt and pepper.
Cut the haddock into 2 pieces and add them to pan. Bring
the stock to a boil, reduce the heat, cover and simmer for 10
minutes until the haddock is just cooked and flakes easily
into even-colored flakes when pressed with a knife.

2 Lift the fish out of the pan, draining well, and transfer it to
a plate. Stir the rice then re-cover and simmer for 15–20
minutes until it is tender and most of the stock has been
absorbed by the rice. Stir several times toward the end of
cooking so that the rice does not stick to the pan.

3 Flake the smoked haddock into pieces, discarding the skin
and any bones. Do the same with the smoked mackerel. Stir
into the just-cooked rice, add the eggs and serve with torn
cilantro leaves scattered over the top.

Nutrition
Wheat and gluten free, low fat
Kcals 357
Fat 16 g
Saturated fat 4 g
Sodium 278 mg
Fiber 2 g

Preparation time
15 minutes
Cooking time
30 minutes
Serves
4

 NUTRITIONAL TIP
If you are avoiding dairy products, omit
the pesto and add some torn basil leaves
and a drizzle of olive oil to the chicken.

chicken en papillotte

Forget about lots of washing up, these tasty chicken parcels, flavored with garlic, pesto, and sun-dried tomatoes, are baked in foil packages, which can be thrown away after use.

10 oz baby new potatoes, scrubbed and sliced

5 oz zucchini, sliced

4 oz mushrooms, sliced

1½ oz sun-dried tomatoes in oil, drained and sliced

salt and pepper

4 boneless, skinless chicken breasts, each about 5 oz

4 teaspoons pesto

2 small garlic cloves, finely chopped (optional)

½ small red onion, thinly sliced

1¼ cups hot gluten- and wheat-free chicken stock or red or white wine

basil leaves, to garnish (optional)

1 Cook the potatoes in a small saucepan of boiling water for 5 minutes until just cooked. Drain.

2 Fold up the edges of 4 large pieces of foil to make 4 containers and put them in a large roasting pan. Spoon the potatoes onto the foil and top with the zucchini, mushroom, and tomato slices. Season lightly with salt and pepper, then top each with a chicken breast.

3 Add a teaspoon of pesto to the top of each chicken breast, sprinkle with the garlic (if used) and red onion and pour the stock around the chicken. Fold the foil over the top of the chicken and twist the edges together to seal well.

4 Bake in a preheated oven, 425°F, for 25 minutes or until the chicken is cooked through and the juices run clear when pierced with a small knife. Transfer the contents of the parcels to serving plates and serve garnished with basil leaves, if desired.

Nutrition

Low fiber

Kcals 283

Fat 13 g

Saturated fat 3 g

Sodium 730 mg

Fiber 1 g

Preparation time

25 minutes

Cooking time

20–25 minutes

Serves

4

NUTRITIONAL TIP

Check the black olive pesto is milk free to enjoy this dish on a milk-free diet.

cod in prosciutto

This stylish-looking supper dish can be prepared in advance and kept in the refrigerator until you are ready to bake it.

2 cod loins, about 1¼ lb in total, rinsed, drained, and each halved crosswise

juice of 1 lemon

salt and pepper

4 teaspoons black olive tapenade or black olive pesto

4 slices prosciutto, about 4 oz in total

1 tablespoon olive oil

1 small onion, finely chopped

1 garlic clove, finely chopped

1 lb plum tomatoes, skinned, seeded, and diced, or 13 oz can chopped tomatoes

2 teaspoons sun-dried tomato paste

2 teaspoons balsamic vinegar (optional)

small bunch of basil

crusty bread, to serve

1 Drizzle the halved fish loins with lemon juice and season, then spread the top and sides with tapenade or pesto, avoiding the ends of the fish. Wrap the top and sides with prosciutto, leaving the ends exposed.

2 Heat the oil in a saucepan, add the onion and garlic and fry for 5 minutes or until softened and lightly browned. Mix in the tomatoes, tomato paste, vinegar (if used), and salt and pepper. Tear the basil leaves into the sauce.

3 Spoon the sauce into a shallow, ovenproof dish and arrange the fish on top. Bake, uncovered, in a preheated oven, 375°F, for 15 minutes until the prosciutto has darkened slightly and the fish is pure white and flakes easily when pressed with a knife. Transfer to plates and serve with crusty bread and rice or new potatoes.

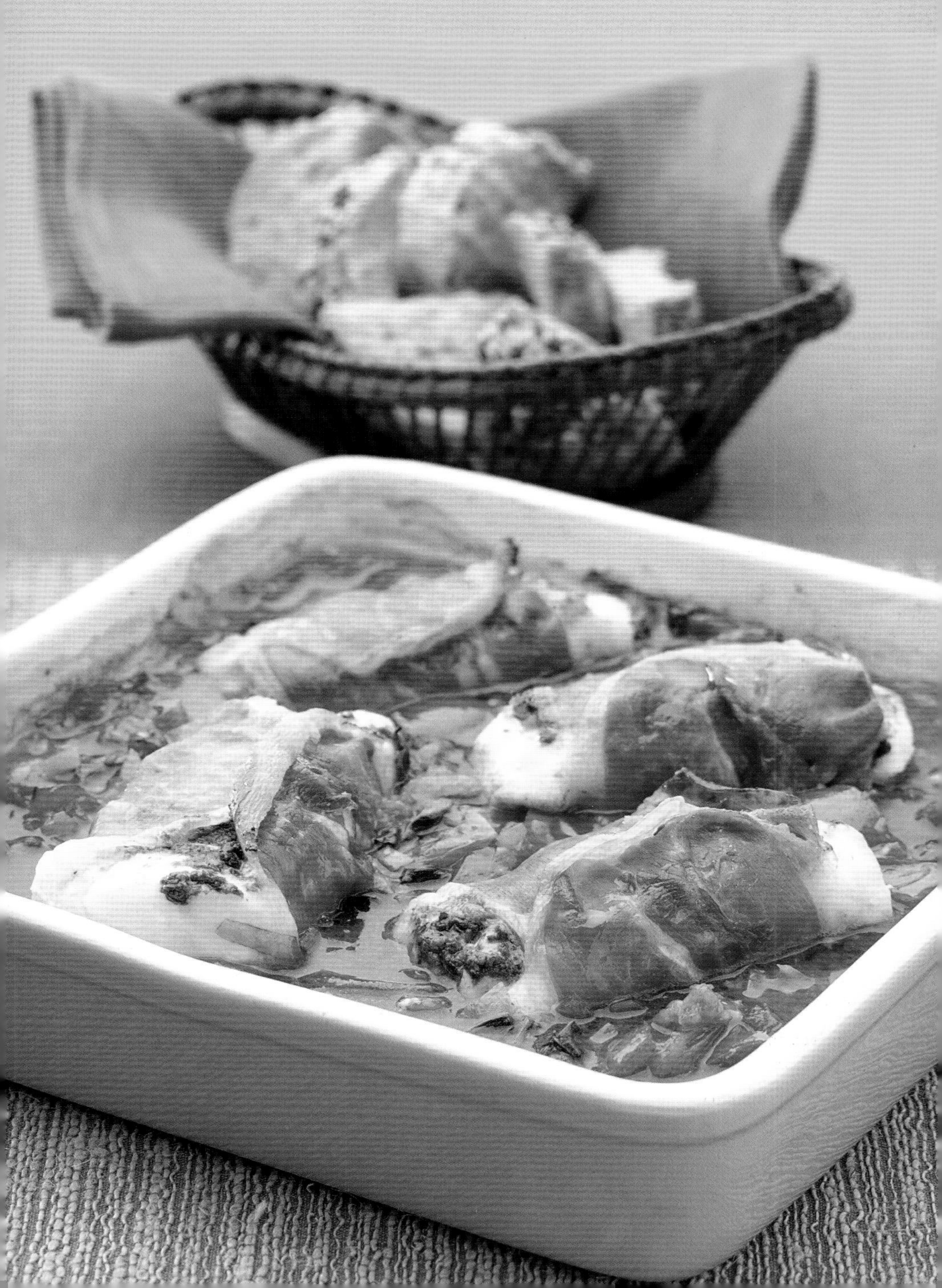

Nutrition

Wheat, gluten and dairy free

Kcals 315

Fat 10 g

Saturated fat 3 g

Sodium 114 mg

Fiber 4 g

Preparation time

15 minutes

Cooking time

2 hours

Serves

4

NUTRITIONAL TIP

Some people with IBS can find beef rather indigestible, but long, slow cooking seems to help. If you do have trouble with it, try not to eat red meat more than once a week and keep the portions small.

peppered beef

This hearty and warming supper can be put on to cook, leaving you free to do other things. If you get delayed the beef will still be fine after 2 hours.

1 tablespoon olive oil

1¼ lb well-trimmed stewing beef, diced

1 onion, roughly chopped

1 garlic clove, finely chopped (optional)

2 tablespoons gluten- and wheat-free white bread flour

2½ cups wheat- and gluten-free beef stock

1 tablespoon tomato paste

1 teaspoon juniper berries, roughly crushed

1 teaspoon peppercorns, roughly crushed

1 bay leaf

½ cup ready-to-eat prunes, pitted and halved

salt

1 Heat the oil in a large skillet, add the beef, a few pieces at a time, until all the pieces have been added to the pan. Add the onion and fry, stirring, over a high heat until the meat is browned and the onion is just beginning to brown.

2 Stir in the garlic (if used) and the flour, then mix in the stock, tomato paste, juniper berries, peppercorns, bay leaf, and prunes. Season with salt and bring to a boil, stirring.

3 Transfer the mixture to a casserole dish, cover and cook in a preheated oven, 325°F, for 2 hours or until the beef is tender. Serve with sweet potato or celeriac mash and green beans.

Nutritional value

Gluten free, high fibre

Kcals 470

Fat 17 g

Saturated fat 7 g

Sodium 433 mg

Fiber 8 g

Preparation time

30 minutes

Cooking time

35 minutes

Serves

4

NUTRITIONAL TIP

If you prefer a thicker sauce, mix with a little water 1 tablespoon of cornstarch or arrowroot and stir into the sauce at the end. If you are avoiding wheat and gluten, check the ingredients list on the mustard, bouillon cubes, and cornstarch before use.

hen house pie

Packed with moist pieces of chicken and lots of fresh vegetables, this pie is topped with cheesy leek and potato mash. It's a perfect supper to enjoy curled up in front of a movie on television.

8 chicken thighs, about 2 lb in total

1 tablespoon olive oil

2 slices of Canadian bacon, diced

2 leeks, about 7 oz in total, thinly sliced

2½ cups wheat- and gluten-free chicken stock

1 teaspoon Dijon mustard

2 tablespoons chopped sage

2 carrots, about 8 oz in total, diced

salt and pepper

1¾ lb potatoes, peeled and diced

7 oz zucchini, diced

1 cup frozen peas

4 tablespoons plain lowfat yogurt

2 oz mature cheddar cheese, grated

1 Cut the skin away from the chicken thighs, cut the meat off the bones and cut it into chunks.

2 Heat the oil in a large skillet, add the chicken a few pieces at a time until it has all been added, then add the bacon and white leek slices. Fry for 5 minutes, stirring until lightly browned. Add 2 cups stock, the mustard, half the sage, and the carrots. Season to taste with salt and pepper, bring to a boil, cover and simmer for 25 minutes.

3 Meanwhile, cook the potatoes until tender, add the green leek slices and cook for 3 minutes more.

4 Add the zucchini, peas, and remaining stock to the chicken mixture and simmer for 5 minutes. Transfer to a shallow, ovenproof dish.

5 Drain the potatoes and leeks and mash them with the yogurt, remaining sage, half the cheese, and season. Spoon over the chicken mixture and sprinkle with the remaining cheese. Put under a preheated broiler until the cheese is bubbling. Serve immediately.

Nutrition
High fiber, wheat free
Kcals 478
Fat 17 g
Saturated fat 6 g
Sodium 200 mg
Fiber 4 g

Preparation time
30 minutes
Cooking time
20 minutes
Serves
4

NUTRITIONAL TIP
Pork tenderloin is low in fat so is much easier to digest than a more traditional lamb or beef roast.

tamarind roasted pork

A stylish roast that is full of flavor. Tamarind has a distinctive, rather sour flavor, and the paste is made from the dried pod of the tamarind tree, shaped into blocks. It is used as a souring agent in many Southeast Asian dishes.

1 tablespoon olive oil

4 teaspoons tamarind paste

1 garlic clove, finely chopped

salt and pepper

4 pieces of pork tenderloin, each 6 oz and 4 inches long

1¼ lb sweet potato, peeled, cut into chunks

2 tablespoons plain yogurt

SALSA
1 dessert apple, cored, diced

½ red onion, finely chopped

½ teaspoon fennel seeds

2 tablespoons cider vinegar

1 teaspoon honey

1 Put the oil, tamarind paste, garlic, and salt and pepper in a plastic bag, add the pieces of pork and toss together until the meat is coated. Transfer to a roasting pan and cook in a preheated oven, 375°F, for about 15 minutes until browned and cook through.

2 Meanwhile, steam the sweet potato for 15–20 minutes or until tender. Take the pork out of the oven, wrap it in foil and allow to rest for 5 minutes.

3 Make the salsa. Place all the ingredients into a small saucepan, cover and simmer for 3–4 minutes or until warmed through.

4 Mash the sweet potato with the yogurt and a little salt and pepper and spoon onto the center of 4 serving plates. Slice the pork thinly and arrange the slices on top of the mash. Serve with green beans, a spoonful of the salsa with the remainder in a small bowl, and the meat juices from the roasting pan drizzled around.

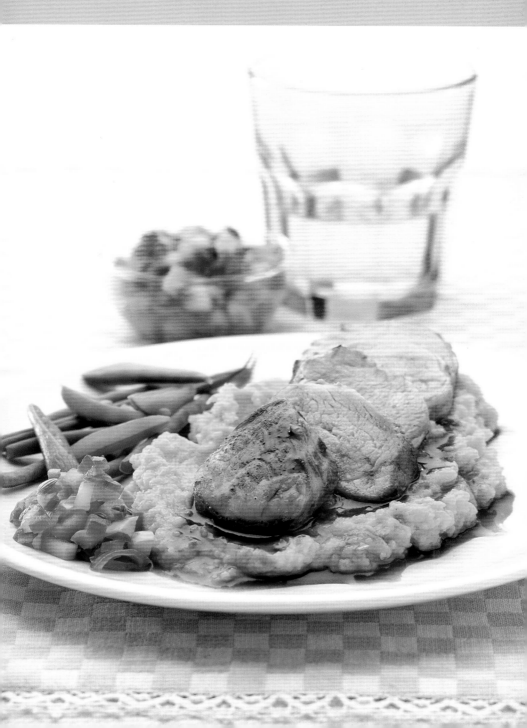

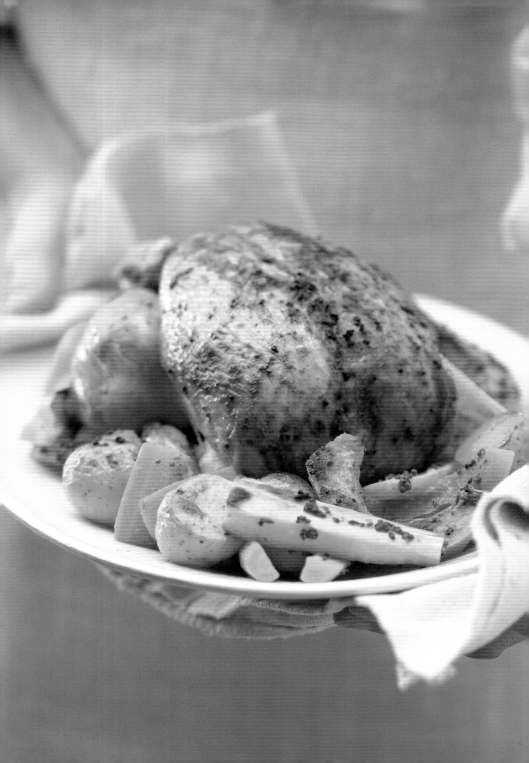

Nutrition

Wheat, gluten free and milk free

Kcals 610

Fat 34 g

Saturated fat 8 g

Sodium 270 mg

Fiber 6 g

Preparation time

25 minutes

Cooking time

1 hour 20 minutes

Serves

4

 NUTRITIONAL TIP

Carefully read the label on the back of the mustard and the bouillon cubes to make sure that they really are gluten free, because some brands may contain wheat flour.

roasted mustard chicken

Glazing the chicken with a mix of honey, wholegrain mustard, and spices means that it cooks to a deep burnished gold. Serve the chicken on its own with the roasted roots or accompany it with a steamed green vegetable.

1 chicken, about 3 lb

3 tablespoons sunflower oil

2 teaspoons wholegrain mustard

2 teaspoons honey

½ teaspoon turmeric

½ teaspoon paprika

salt and pepper

½ butternut squash, about 10 oz, peeled and seeded

3 carrots, about 10 oz in total

2 parsnips, about 8 oz in total

10 oz baby new potatoes, scrubbed

1¼ cups chicken or vegetable stock

1 Rinse the chicken inside and out with cold water, drain well and transfer to a large roasting pan.

2 Mix together the oil, mustard, honey, spices, and salt and pepper in a large mixing bowl, then brush a little over the chicken. Loosely cover with oiled foil and roast in a preheated oven, 375°F, for 30 minutes.

3 Meanwhile, cut the flesh of the butternut squash into thick slices. Cut the carrots and parsnips into chunky sticks. Halve any large potatoes.

4 Remove the foil from the chicken and brush with some more mustard mixture. Add the vegetables to the remaining mustard mix and toss together in the bowl. Spoon around the chicken and roast for 50 minutes, turning once or twice and re-covering the chicken after 20–30 minutes or when the skin is deep brown.

5 Insert a skewer through the thickest part of the chicken leg into the breast. If the juices run clear, transfer the chicken and vegetables to a serving plate. If not, return to the oven and retest after 15 minutes. Pour off half the fat from the roasting pan, add the stock to the remaining juices, bring to a boil, and strain into a pitcher before serving.

Nutrition	Preparation time	NUTRITIONAL TIP
Wheat free, gluten free	15 minutes	If you are on a dairy-free diet, omit the
Kcals 319	**Cooking time**	yogurt altogether or use soy yogurt
Fat 18 g	about 1 hour	instead.
Saturated fat 8 g	10 minutes	
Sodium 185 mg	**Serves**	
Fiber 3 g	4	

spicy lamb with eggplant

This dish has all the flavor of a Greek moussaka but none of the fiddle. If you prefer not to serve it with rice, it would taste delicious topped with mashed potato mixed with lowfat yogurt rather than butter and milk and browned in the oven.

1 tablespoon olive oil

1 onion, chopped

1 lb lean lamb, ground

1 eggplant, about 8 oz, halved lengthwise and thinly sliced

1–2 garlic cloves, finely chopped

13 oz can chopped tomatoes

1 teaspoon ground cinnamon

¼ teaspoon grated nutmeg

1¼ cups wheat- and gluten-free lamb or chicken stock

salt and pepper

4 tablespoons Greek or whole milk yogurt, to serve

roughly chopped mint or flat-leaf parsley, to serve

paprika (optional)

1 Heat the oil in a flameproof casserole, add the onion and lamb and fry for 2 minutes. Add the eggplant and fry for 5 minutes or until the lamb is evenly browned and the onion and eggplant are softened.

2 Stir in the garlic, tomatoes, spices, stock, and a little salt and pepper. Bring to the boil, stirring, and cover.

3 Cook the lamb mixture in a preheated oven, 350°F, for 1 hour or until tender. Serve with rice and topped with a spoonful of yogurt and sprinkled with mint, parsley, and paprika, if desired.

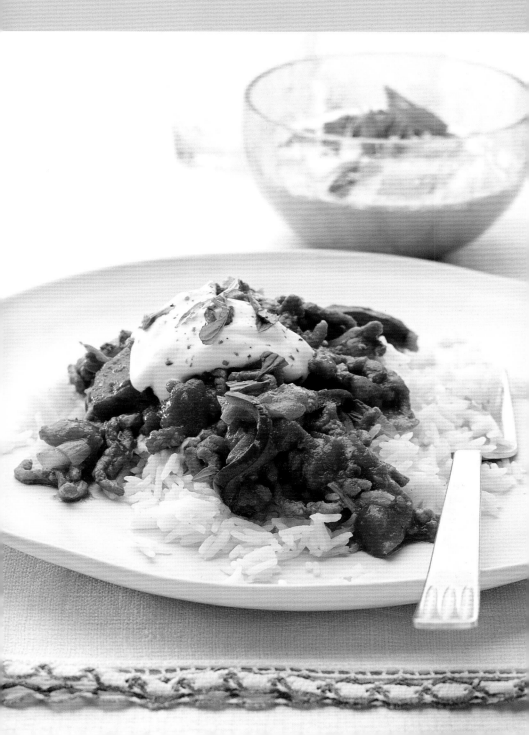

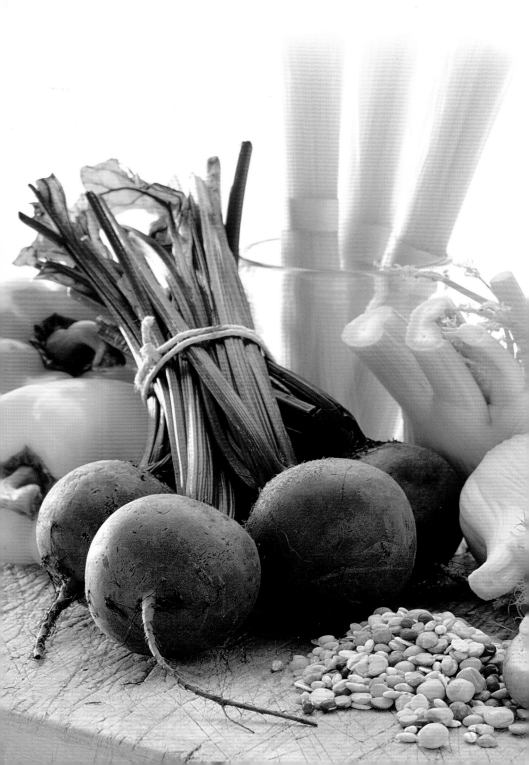

vegetarian

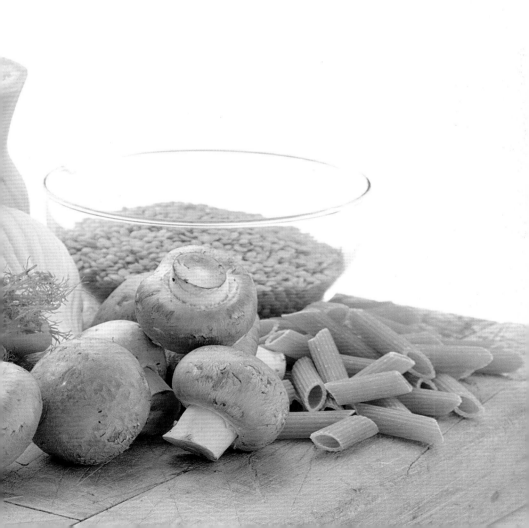

Nutrition
Wheat and gluten free, high fiber
Kcals 380
Fat 15 g
Saturated fat 7 g
Sodium 357 mg
Fiber 4 g

Preparation time
15 minutes
Cooking time
about 30 minutes
Serves
4

NUTRITIONAL TIP
If you cannot tolerate dairy products, omit
the cheese. Check that the cheese you are
using is suitable for vegetarians and is not
made with rennet.

beet and blue cheese risotto

A vibrant red, soft, and creamy risotto is speckled with just-melting blue cheese.
Serve as soon as the rice is cooked or the liquid will quickly be absorbed because the
rice swells on standing. If you're not a fan of blue cheese, add a little freshly grated
Parmesan instead.

1 tablespoon olive oil

1 onion, finely chopped

**3 small uncooked beets,
trimmed weight about 12 oz,
peeled and diced**

1 cup arborio rice

salt and pepper

**few sage leaves, plus extra
to garnish**

**5 cups hot wheat- and gluten-
free vegetable stock**

**4 oz St Agur, Stilton, or other
blue cheese, rind removed,
and diced**

1 Heat the oil in a nonstick skillet, add the onion and fry
gently, stirring occasionally, for 5 minutes or until softened.
Stir in the beet and cook for 2 minutes.

2 Stir in the rice, then add the sage, a little salt and pepper,
and about one-third of the hot stock. Simmer, uncovered, for
15–20 minutes until the rice is soft and creamy and the beet
is tender, topping up with the remaining stock and stirring
more frequently toward the end of cooking.

3 Stir in the cheese and sprinkle with extra sage leaves,
if desired. Spoon into bowls and serve immediately.

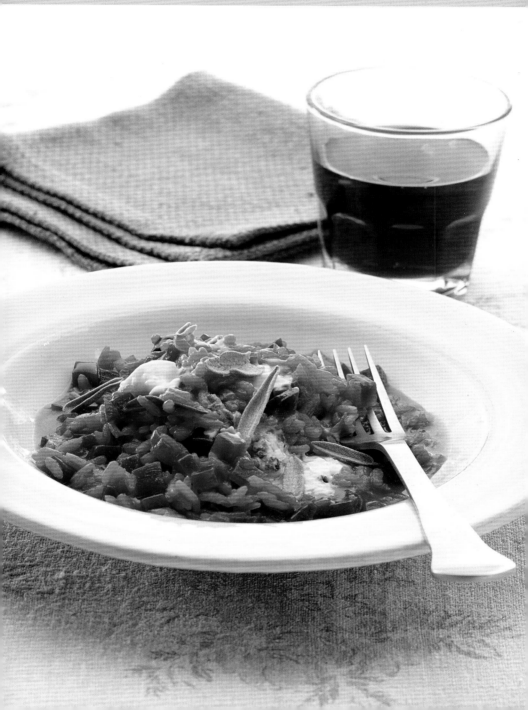

Nutrition
Wheat, gluten and dairy free
Kcals 340
Fat 13 g
Saturated fat 3 g
Sodium 513 mg
Fiber 4 g

Preparation time
20 minutes
Cooking time
about 30 minutes
Serves
4

NUTRITIONAL TIP
The fiber content of the dish will vary depending on the vegetable you choose and the type of rice. To reduce the fiber level, use white rice.

special fried rice

Popular with all ages, this tasty supper can be made with whatever vegetables you have in the refrigerator. Just take care that you cut them into small pieces so that they cook quickly.

1 cup easy-cook brown rice

3 eggs

1 tablespoon water

salt and pepper

6 teaspoons sunflower oil

4 scallions, sliced

4 oz zucchini, diced

½ red bell pepper, cored, seeded, and diced

2 oz snow peas, sliced

¾ cup frozen peas

1 inch ginger root, peeled and grated

2 tablespoons sesame seeds

2 tablespoons tamari sauce

1 Cook the rice in boiling water for about 25 minutes or according to the instructions on the package until just tender.

2 Meanwhile, beat together the eggs, water, and a little salt and pepper in a bowl. Heat 2 teaspoons oil in a large skillet, add the eggs and make a thin omelet. When the underside is golden, turn it over and cook the other side for a minute more. Slide it out of pan onto a plate and set aside.

3 Heat 3 teaspoons oil in the skillet, then add the scallions, zucchini, bell pepper, snow peas, peas and ginger. Stir-fry for 3–4 minutes or until tender. Drain the rice, tip it back into the dried pan, and stir in the stir-fried vegetables.

4 Heat the remaining oil in a skillet, add the sesame seeds and fry for 2–3 minutes, stirring until just beginning to brown. Turn off the heat, add the tamari sauce and quickly cover the pan so that the seeds do not ping out.

5 Roll up the omelet, cut it into thin slices and add to the rice with the sesame seeds. Spoon into bowls and serve.

Nutrition

Wheat and gluten free, high fiber

Kcals 533

Fat 16 g

Saturated fat 2 g

Sodium 860 mg

Fiber 4 g

Preparation time

15 minutes

Cooking time

8–10 minutes

Serves

4

NUTRITIONAL TIP

Use soy yogurt in the tzatziki to make this dish suitable for a dairy-free diet.

falafel

These chickpea patties are traditionally deep-fried, but this pan-fried version is healthier. Made in minutes using a can of chickpeas, falafel are packed with protein and fiber.

1 onion, quartered

small bunch of parsley or chives

2 garlic cloves, sliced

2 x 13¼ oz cans chickpeas, drained

2 teaspoons cumin seeds, finely crushed

2 teaspoons coriander seeds, finely crushed

1 teaspoon wheat- and gluten-free baking powder

3 tablespoons olive oil

salt and pepper

TZATZIKI
4 oz cucumber, finely diced

⅔ cup lowfat plain yogurt

few fresh mint leaves

4 pita breads, to serve

2 crisphead lettuce leaves, to serve

1 Put all the ingredients for the falafel into a food processor and blend to make a coarse, thick puree. Alternatively, blend in batches or finely chop the onion, herbs, garlic, and chickpeas and mix them with the remaining ingredients.

2 Use 2 dessertspoons to shape the mixture into 16 oval patties. Heat 1 tablespoon oil in a large, nonstick skillet, add half the falafel and fry for 4–5 minutes, turning until golden and crisp on the outside and piping hot. Add extra oil if needed. Repeat with the remaining falafel.

3 Meanwhile, make the tzatziki by mixing together the cucumber, yogurt and mint in a bowl. Warm the pita breads under the broiler and shred the lettuce if desired. Arrange on serving plates with the hot falafel.

Nutrition
Wheat and gluten free, high fiber
Kcals 285
Fat 10 g
Saturated fat 4 g
Sodium 413 mg
Fiber 5 g

Preparation time
25 minutes
Cooking time
about 1 hour
10 minutes
Serves
4

 NUTRITIONAL TIP
If you are avoiding wheat and gluten and
are not on a dairy-free diet, omit the toast
and add some sliced cheese once the
ratatouille has been served. You could also
serve this with baked potato, rice, or pasta.

oven-baked ratatouille

Florence fennel adds a delicate aniseed flavor to this rich ratatouille, which is
speckled with bell peppers and zucchini and topped with toasted baguette slices
and creamy, just-melting goat cheese with chives.

1 tablespoon olive oil

1 onion, chopped

2 garlic cloves, finely chopped

1 fennel bulb, about 8 oz, diced

3 colored bell peppers, cored,
seeded, and diced

2 zucchini, about 10 oz
in total, diced

13 oz can chopped tomatoes

²⁄₃ cup wheat- and gluten-free
vegetable stock

1 teaspoon superfine sugar

salt and pepper

arugula salad, to serve

TOPPING
1 baguette, about 5 oz in total,
thinly sliced

4 oz goat cheese
with chives

1 Heat the oil in a large, nonstick skillet. Add the onion and
fry, stirring, for 5 minutes or until lightly browned. Add the
garlic and remaining fresh vegetables and fry for an
additional 2 minutes.

2 Stir in the canned tomatoes, stock, sugar, and a little salt
and pepper. Bring to a boil, stirring, then transfer to a deep
ovenproof dish. Cover the top of the dish with foil and bake
in a preheated oven, 375°F, for 45–60 minutes until the
vegetables are tender.

3 When the vegetables are almost ready, broil one side of
the bread slices. Slice the cheese and add one slice to each
untoasted side of bread. Remove the foil from the ratatouille,
stir the vegetables and top with the toasts, cheese side up.

4 Put the ratatouille under a preheated broiler for
4–5 minutes until the cheese is just beginning to melt.
Spoon into shallow bowls and serve with an arugula salad.

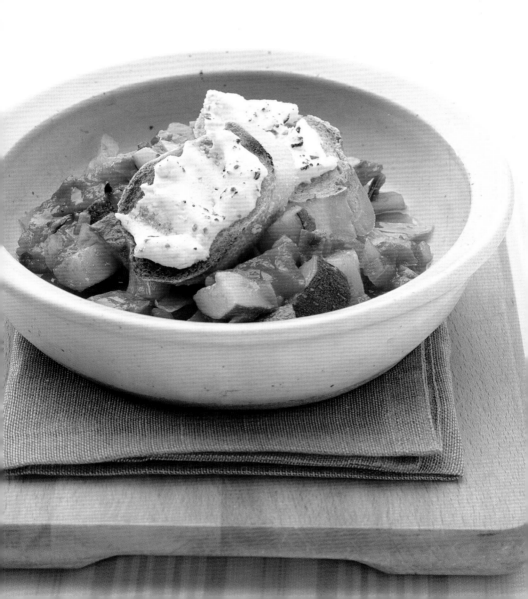

Nutrition
Dairy free, high fiber
Kcals 305
Fat 5 g
Saturated fat 1 g
Sodium 47 mg
Fiber 5 g

Preparation time
15 minutes
Cooking time
30 minutes
Serves
4

NUTRITIONAL TIP
Spicy foods can upset IBS. Choosing milder spices or cutting the amount used may help.

bulgar pilaf with mixed roots

An easy pantry supper, this can be served as it is or topped with spoonfuls of yogurt, toasted nuts, or torn mint or parsley leaves. Cut the vegetables into small dice so that they cook quickly.

1 tablespoon olive oil

1 red onion, sliced

²/₃ cup diced parsnip

1¹/₃ cups diced carrot

1¹/₂ cups diced rutabaga

4 cloves

1 teaspoon ground cinnamon

1 teaspoon mild paprika

½ teaspoon ground cumin

13¹/₄ oz can green lentils, drained

³/₄ cup bulgar wheat

1 tablespoon tomato paste

salt and pepper

about 4 cups vegetable stock

1 Heat the oil in a large, nonstick skillet, add the onion and fry, stirring, for 5 minutes or until softened. Stir in the root vegetables and fry for 2 minutes.

2 Mix in the spices, cook for an additional minute, then add the lentils, bulgar wheat, tomato paste, and a little salt and pepper. Pour in 2¹/₂ cups stock and bring to a boil.

3 Reduce the heat, cover and simmer for 20 minutes, stirring and topping up with extra stock as needed, until the vegetables are tender. Spoon into bowls to serve.

Nutrition

Wheat, gluten and dairy free

Kcals 389

Fat 20 g

Saturated fat 8 g

Sodium 614 g

Fiber 2 g

Preparation time

10 minutes

Cooking time

10 minutes

Serves

4

NUTRITIONAL TIP

The fiber content of this dish will depend on the vegetables you use, so you can adjust the recipe for either a high- or a low-fiber diet.

mixed vegetable and cashew laska

This light, refreshing, and colorful curry can be cooked in under 10 minutes. Vary the vegetables depending on what you have in the refrigerator.

4 oz medium rice noodles

2 teaspoons sunflower oil

1 onion, finely chopped

½ cup cashew nuts

2 teaspoons wheat- and gluten-free red Thai curry paste

1 garlic clove, finely chopped

14 fl oz can reduced-fat coconut milk

1¼ cups wheat- and gluten-free vegetable stock

4 oz carrot, cut into matchstick strips

1 red bell pepper, cored, seeded, and diced

2 oz snow peas, sliced

4 oz bok choy, sliced

2 tablespoons tamari sauce

small bunch of basil or fresh cilantro

1 Cook the noodles in boiling water according to the instructions on the package.

2 Meanwhile, heat the oil in a wok or second saucepan, add the onion and cashew nuts and fry for 3–4 minutes until just beginning to brown. Stir in the curry paste and garlic, then mix in the coconut milk and stock.

3 Bring the coconut broth to a boil, add the carrot and red pepper and simmer for 3 minutes. Mix in the snow peas and bok choy and cook for an additional 2 minutes until the leaves have just wilted. Stir in the tamari sauce and half the basil or cilantro, torn into pieces.

4 Drain the noodles and stir them into the coconut broth. Spoon into bowls and top with the remaining basil or cilantro leaves.

Nutrition
High fiber
Kcals 404
Fat 11 g
Saturated fat 3 g
Sodium 33 mg
Fiber 11 g

Preparation time
15 minutes
Cooking time
15 minutes
Serves
4

NUTRITIONAL TIP
Reduce the fat content even more by
using lowfat ricotta instead of the yogurt.
If you are avoiding dairy products, omit
the yogurt altogether.

penne with roasted tomatoes

Whole-wheat pasta has been used here, but plain pasta or corn pasta can be used
instead. Alternatively, spoon the tomato sauce over the top of a baked potato.

1 lb cherry tomatoes, halved

2 tablespoons olive oil

2 garlic cloves, finely chopped

4–5 stems rosemary

large pinch of smoked paprika
or chili powder

salt and pepper

12 oz dried whole-wheat pasta
twists or tubes

2 tablespoons balsamic vinegar

4 tablespoons plain yogurt

Parmesan shavings, to serve

1 Put the tomatoes in a roasting pan, drizzle with the oil and
sprinkle with the garlic, torn leaves from 3 rosemary stems,
the paprika or chili powder, and a little salt and pepper. Roast
in a preheated oven, 400°F, for 15 minutes until just softened.

2 Meanwhile, cook the pasta in a large saucepan of boiling
water for 10–12 minutes or until just tender, then drain.

3 Spoon the balsamic vinegar into the tomatoes, add the
drained pasta and yogurt and lightly toss together. Spoon
into bowls and top with Parmesan shavings.

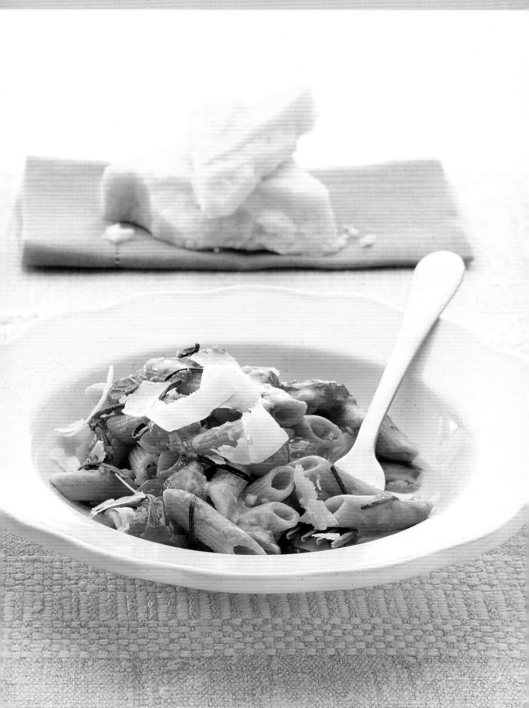

Nutrition
Wheat, gluten and dairy free
Kcals 186
Fat 12 g
Saturated fat 3 g
Sodium 118 mg
Fiber 1 g

Preparation time
10 minutes
Cooking time
12–14 minutes
Serves
4

✚ **NUTRITIONAL TIP**
Increase the fiber levels by adding frozen peas or frozen fava beans together with the diced zucchini.

minted zucchini frittata

A quick and easy summer supper, this is even easier if you have fresh mint growing in your garden. If you don't have any fresh herbs use a little chopped watercress or arugula leaves or some frozen parsley. If you like, add some diced chorizo, bacon, salami or ham, or extra vegetables when you fry the zucchini.

4 teaspoons olive oil

1 red onion, thinly sliced

12 oz zucchini, diced

6 eggs

2 tablespoons water

2 tablespoons chopped mint

salt and pepper

mixed salad, to serve

1 Heat 3 teaspoons oil in a large, nonstick skillet, add the onion and zucchini and fry over a gentle heat for 5 minutes or until lightly browned and just cooked.

2 Beat together the eggs, water, chopped mint, and a little salt and pepper. Heat the remaining oil in the skillet and pour in the egg mixture. Cook, without stirring, for 4–5 minutes or until the frittata is almost set and the underside is golden-brown.

3 Transfer the pan to a hot broiler (making sure that the handle is away from the heat) and cook for 3–4 minutes until the top is golden and the frittata is cooked through. Cut into wedges or squares and serve with a mixed salad.

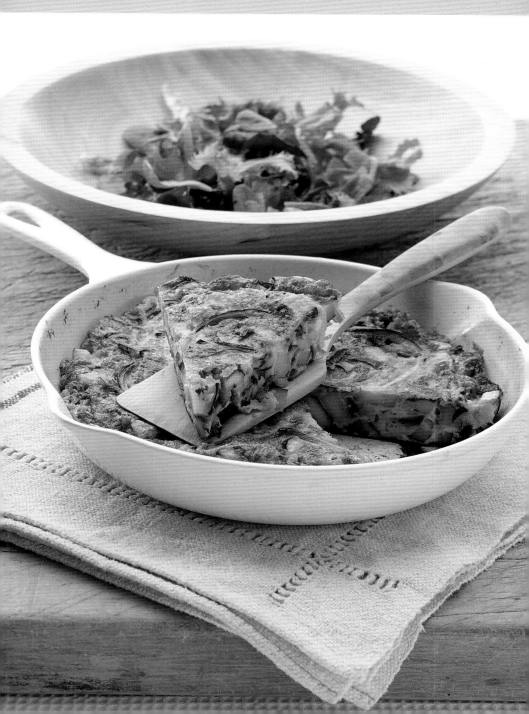

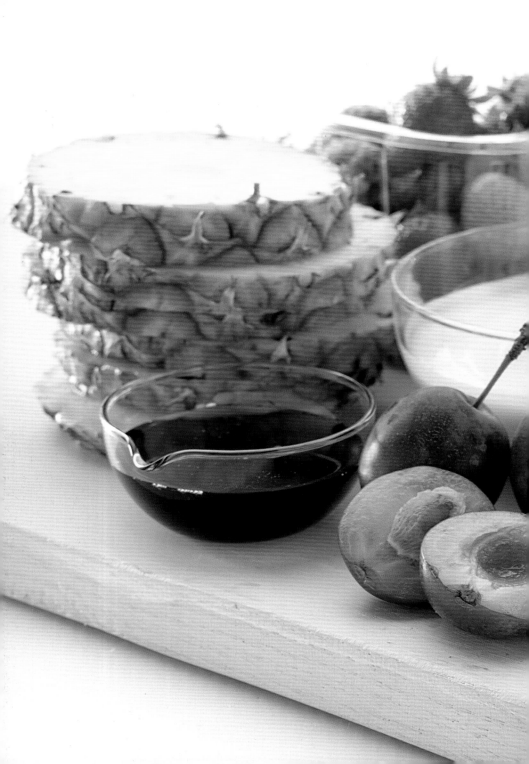

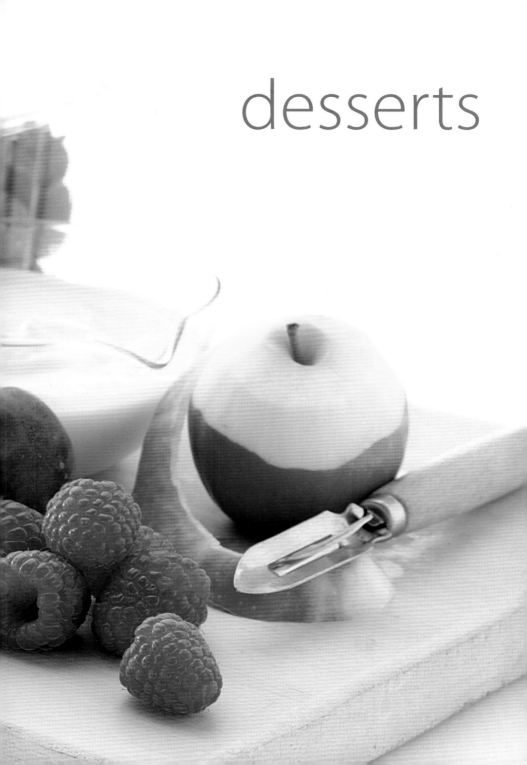

desserts

Nutrition
Wheat and gluten free, low fiber
Kcals 125
Fat 2 g (1 g fat per 100 g)
Saturated fat 1 g
Sodium 33 mg
Fiber 2 g

Preparation time
15 minutes
Cooking time
15 minutes
Serves
4

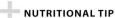 **NUTRITIONAL TIP**
If you are not on a dairy-free diet, serve
the peaches with scoops of vanilla ice
cream. Make sure you use chocolate with
70 percent cocoa solids if you are avoiding
milk and check the ingredients list to make
sure it is dairy free.

peach melba meringues

When you're short of time but really want to make a pudding to impress your friends,
this is the answer. Halved and baked peaches are topped with a square of melting
chocolate and a soft-centered marshmallow meringue topping before being
drizzled with a ruby-red fresh raspberry sauce.

**2 large peaches, halved
and pitted**

**4 squares of dark chocolate,
about 1 oz**

2 egg whites

¼ cup superfine sugar

**2 cups raspberries (just thawed
if frozen)**

**a little sifted confectioners'
sugar, to decorate (optional)**

1 Put the peaches, cut side up, in a shallow ovenproof dish,
add 2 tablespoons water to the base of the dish and cover
the peaches loosely with foil. Bake in a preheated oven,
350°F, for 10 minutes.

2 Add a square of chocolate to the center of each peach half,
re-cover and return to the oven.

3 Meanwhile, make the meringue. Beat the egg whites until
they form stiff but moist-looking peaks. Gradually beat in
the sugar, a teaspoonful at a time, until the mixture is thick
and glossy.

4 Spoon the meringue over the peaches and swirl into
peaks with the back of the spoon. Return the peaches to the
oven for 5–7 minutes until the meringue is cooked through
and the swirls are tinged with brown.

5 Meanwhile, puree 1 cup of the raspberries and sieve to
remove the seeds. Transfer the peaches to serving plates,
decorate with the remaining whole raspberries, drizzle the
sauce around and dust with sifted confectioners' sugar, if
desired. Serve immediately.

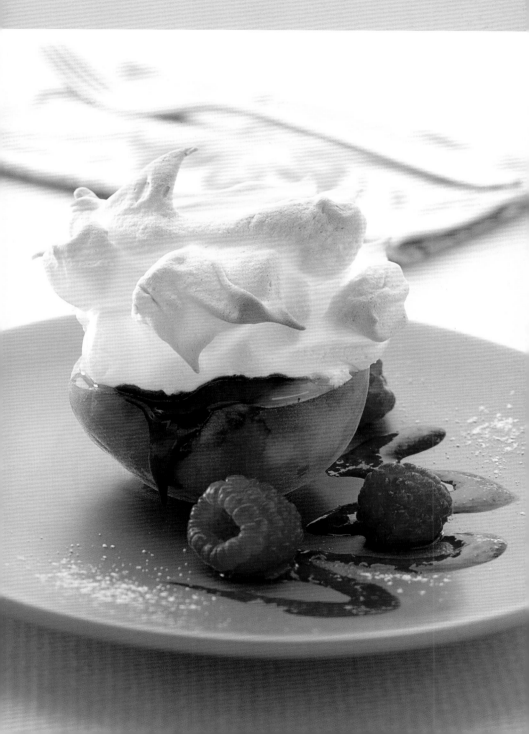

Nutrition
Wheat, gluten and dairy free
Kcals 249
Fat 9 g
Saturated fat 6 g
Sodium 120 mg
Fiber 3 g

Preparation time
20–30 minutes, plus
freezing
Cooking time
none
Serves
4

NUTRITIONAL TIP
This is much lower in sugar and fat than
a more conventional dairy ice cream.

lychee and coconut ice

This dairy-free ice cream tastes delicious when it is used to sandwich tiny pairs of
spooned or piped meringues. If you make the ice cream in advance, leave it at room
temperature for about 15 minutes to soften slightly before scooping.

**14 oz can lychees in natural
syrup**

½ cup icing sugar

grated zest of 2 limes

**14 fl oz can reduced-fat
coconut milk**

3 cups strawberries

1 Put the lychees and the juice into a blender or food
processor, reserving 2 for decoration later. Add the
confectioners' sugar and puree until smooth.

2 Stir in the lime zest and coconut milk, then pour into a
chilled ice-cream maker and churn until thick enough to
scoop, which should take about 30 minutes. Alternatively,
pour the mixture into a shallow stainless-steel roasting pan
and freeze for 4–6 hours, beating 2–3 times with a fork or
blitzing in a food processor to break down the ice crystals
and returning to the freezer until it is firm enough to scoop.

3 Meanwhile, hull and puree half the strawberries. Sieve to
remove the seeds. Slice or quarter the remaining fruits,
depending on their size.

4 To serve, scoop the coconut ice into glasses, drizzle with
the pureed sauce and top with the remaining berries and
reserved lychees, cut into slices.

Nutrition

Wheat and gluten free, low fat

Kcals 197

Fat 5 g

Saturated fat 3 g

Sodium 68 mg

Fiber 3 g

Preparation time

30 minutes

Cooking time

45 minutes

Serves

4

+ NUTRITIONAL TIP

Some brands of cornstarch contain wheat flour, so read the ingredients list carefully if you are avoiding gluten. To make this suitable for a milk-free diet, use soy cream or yogurt.

brown sugar pavlovas with berries

Don't wait for a special occasion to make this dish. Serve four now and leave the plain pavlovas in an airtight container for up to three days, then just top them with fresh, frozen, or canned fruit as and when you need them.

3 egg whites

½ cup soft light brown sugar

⅓ cup superfine sugar

1 teaspoon gluten-free cornstarch

1 teaspoon white wine vinegar

TO DECORATE
¾ cup reduced-fat sour cream

1¼ cups raspberries (just thawed if frozen)

1½ cups strawberries, sliced

sifted confectioners' sugar (optional)

1 Beat the egg whites until they form stiff but moist-looking peaks. Gradually beat in the sugars, a teaspoonful at a time, and continue to beat for 1–2 minutes or until the egg whites have turned thick and glossy.

2 Mix the cornstarch with the vinegar and fold into the meringue. Grease and line a large baking sheet and spoon the meringue onto the sheet in 6 mounds, spreading it into circles about 4 inches across.

3 Bake the pavlovas in a preheated oven, 275°F, for 35–40 minutes or until crisp on the outside and they can be lifted easily off the paper. Allow to cool.

4 Peel the pavlovas off the paper and transfer them to serving plates. Spoon the sour cream over the top and decorate with the berries. To serve, dust with a little sifted confectioners' sugar, if desired.

Nutrition

Wheat free, high fiber

Kcals 109

Fat 2 g

Saturated fat 1 g

Sodium 73 g

Fiber 7 g

Preparation time

10 minutes

Cooking time

Serves

4

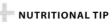 **NUTRITIONAL TIP**

To reduce the fiber content, make up your own bags of fresh strawberries and raspberries only. Soy yogurt will make this dessert suitable for a milk-free and exclusion diet.

cheats' summer berry sundae

This really speedy dessert is made in a matter of seconds and is just bursting with flavor. Crème de cassis could be used in place of the cordial if you prefer, and dainty soft amaretti biscuits or biscotti could be served alongside if you are not avoiding wheat.

3 cups frozen mixed summer berries, partially thawed

3 tablespoons blackcurrant cordial (undiluted)

1 cup lowfat Greek or whole milk yogurt

4 teaspoons honey

2 tablespoons chopped mint

1 Put the fruit and cordial into a food processor or blender and blitz until crushed and sorbet like.

2 Mix the yogurt with the honey and chopped mint. Add alternate spoonfuls of pureed fruit and yogurt to 4 glasses, then swirl together with the handle of a teaspoon to give a marbled effect.

3 Decorate with extra mint leaves or a tiny sprig of mint dusted lightly with sifted confectioners' sugar, if desired.

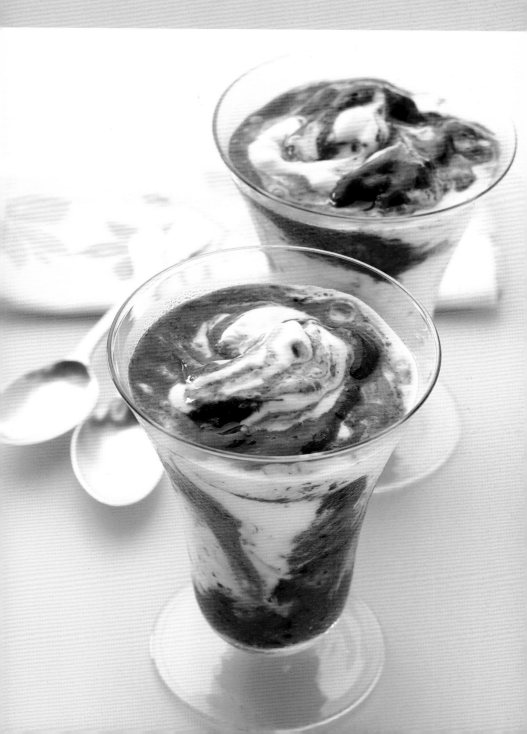

Nutrition

Wheat free, gluten free

Kcals 332

Fat 6 g

Saturated fat 4 g

Sodium 89 mg

Fiber 3 g

Preparation time

20 minutes

Cooking time

40–45 minutes

Serves

4

 NUTRITIONAL TIP

To reduce the fiber level, use white arborio rice and cook for 20 minutes until tender. To lower the fat levels, use reduced-fat yogurt. For a dairy-free version, use soy milk or rice milk to make the risotto. This will make it suitable for an exclusion diet.

red rice risotto with roasted plums

Spoon down through the hot roasted plums to a generous spoonful of sour cream and then into the warmth of the nutty red rice scented with vanilla and cinnamon. Use pitted cherries in season or try stirring a little cocoa powder into the rice along with the sugar for a change.

1 cup red rice

2 cups lowfat milk

2 cups water

¼ teaspoon ground cinnamon, plus extra to sprinkle

8 oz ripe red plums, quartered and pitted

2 tablespoons superfine sugar

1 teaspoon vanilla extract

4 tablespoons reduced-fat sour cream

1 Put the rice, half the milk and water and the cinnamon into a saucepan. Bring to a boil, reduce the heat and simmer for 40–45 minutes, stirring occasionally and topping up with milk and water as needed until the rice is soft and creamy.

2 Toward the end of the cooking time for the rice, put the plums into a shallow, ovenproof dish, sprinkle with a little extra cinnamon and add a tablespoon of water to the base of the dish. Bake in a preheated oven, 350F, for 10 minutes.

3 Stir the sugar and vanilla extract into the rice. Spoon into shallow dishes, top with spoonfuls of sour cream, sprinkle with a little extra cinnamon and arrange the plums to the side of the sour cream.

Nutrition

Wheat, gluten and milk free

Kcals 108

Fat 0 g

Saturated fat 0 g

Sodium 7 mg

Fiber 3 g

Preparation time

10 minutes

Cooking time

15–20 minutes

Serves

4

NUTRITIONAL TIP

If you are not avoiding dairy products, serve the pears with spoonfuls of reduced-fat sour cream, Greek or whole milk yogurt drizzled with a little extra honey. This dish is suitable for an exclusion diet.

saffron and ginger poached pears

Quick and easy to prepare, these light and refreshing poached pears taste just as delicious served warm or chilled. They also freeze well, so why not make up a double quantity in advance of a supper to share with friends?

1 ¼ cups apple juice

2 large pinches of saffron threads

½ inch ginger root, peeled and cut into thin strips

1 tablespoon honey

4 pears, each about 5 oz

1 Put the apple juice, saffron, ginger, and honey into a medium saucepan and heat gently for 5 minutes.

2 Meanwhile, peel the pears, leaving the stalks on, and remove the calyx from the base. Add the pears to the saucepan and press below the surface of the apple juice. (If necessary change to a smaller pan.)

3 Simmer gently for 15–20 minutes, turning the pears occasionally so that they color evenly and are just tender. Spoon into a small pedestal dish and serve warm or chilled.

Nutrition

Low fat, gluten free

Kcals 155

Fat 1 g

Saturated fat 0 g

Sodium 16 mg

Fiber 3 g

Preparation time

10 minutes

Cooking time

4–5 minutes

Serves

4

NUTRITIONAL TIP

Anyone on a milk-free or exclusion diet could use soy yogurt instead of lowfat yogurt.

maple-glazed pineapple

Speedy enough to prepare while someone else clears the main course plates, this colorful dessert is just the thing to make for a last-minute meal to share with friends.

6 slices fresh pineapple, peeled, cored, and halved

¾ cup blueberries

8 teaspoons maple syrup

1 banana, about 7 oz with skin on

⅔ cup lowfat plain yogurt

2 teaspoons chopped crystallized ginger or stem ginger, drained and chopped

1 Arrange the pineapple slices in a single layer on a deep baking sheet. Sprinkle the blueberries over and around the pineapple, then drizzle the pineapple with 4 teaspoons maple syrup.

2 Cook the fruit under a preheated broiler for 4–5 minutes until the pineapple is beginning to brown and the juices have begun to run from the blueberries.

3 Meanwhile, peel and mash the banana and mix it with the yogurt and ginger.

4 Arrange the pineapple on serving plates. Spoon the blueberries and their juices over the top and the banana yogurt to one side. Drizzle with the remaining maple syrup and serve immediately.

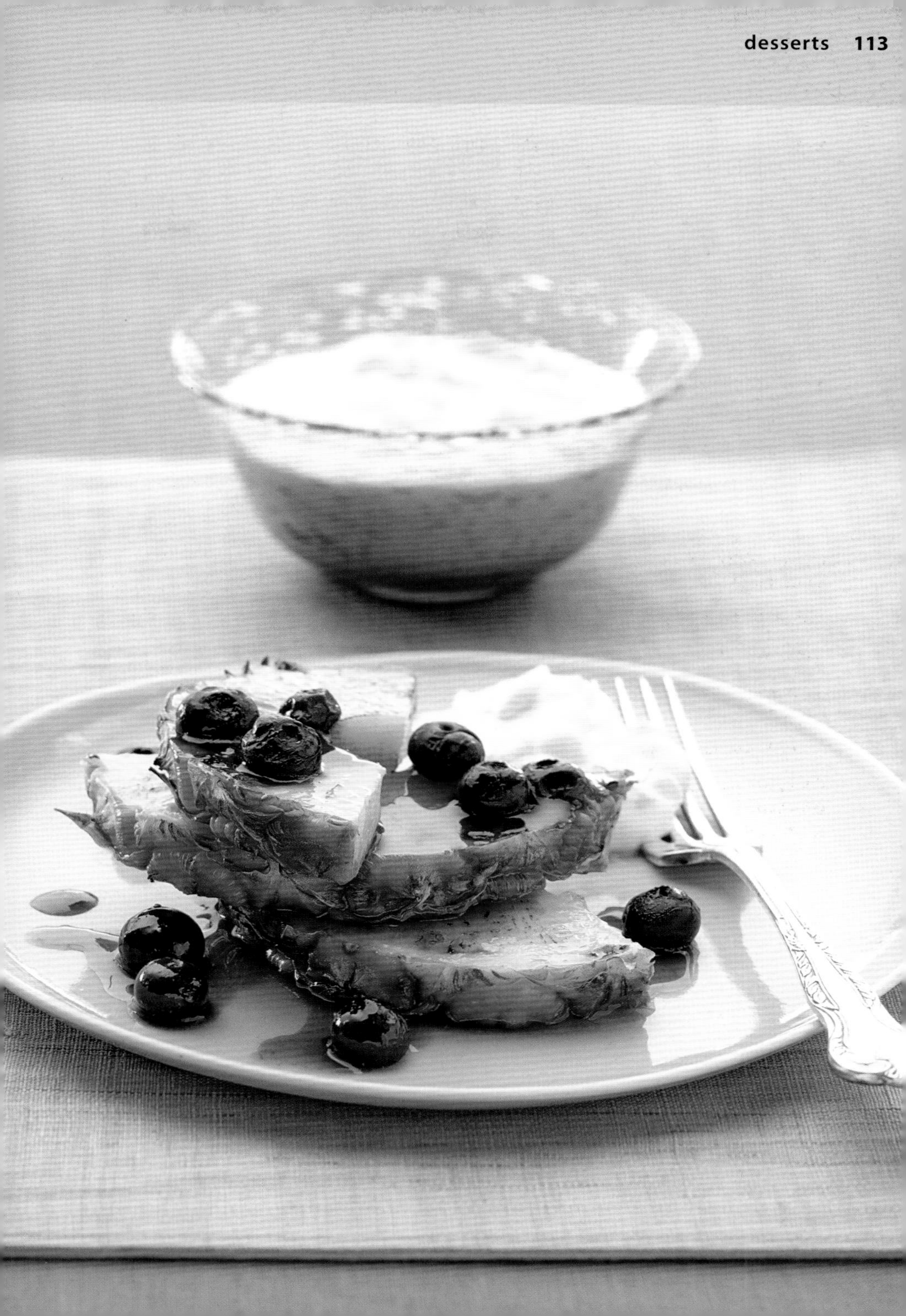

Nutrition
High fiber
Kcals 386
Fat 14 g
Saturated fat 2 g
Sodium 90 mg
Fiber 7 g

Preparation time
20 minutes
Cooking time
25–30 minutes
Serves
4

NUTRITIONAL TIP
If you are avoiding dairy products, use soy margarine and do not serve with custard or ice cream unless made with soy milk. To reduce the fibre content, omit the oats and seeds from the crumble and make up the flour to 100 g (3½ oz).

apple and blackberry oat crumble

A homely pudding, this is perfect after a Sunday roast or slow-cooked casserole. The crumble topping can be made in larger batches and kept in the freezer. Simply sprinkle it over cooked fruits while still frozen and transfer to the oven. You might also like to try this with apples only, plums, or a mix of plums and pears.

2 cooking apples, about 1 lb in total, quartered, cored, and peeled

²/₃ cup blackberries

½ cup soft light brown sugar

¾ cup all-purpose flour

¼ cup reduced-fat spread

⅓ cup rolled oats

2 tablespoons slivered almonds

2 tablespoons sunflower seeds

finely grated zest of ½ small orange

custard or ice cream, to serve

1 Thinly slice the apples and put them in a saucepan with the blackberries, 2 tablespoons sugar and 6 tablespoons water. Cover and simmer for 5 minutes or until partly cooked.

2 Meanwhile, put the remaining sugar in a bowl with the flour. Add the spread and blend in using your fingertips until the mixture resembles fine bread crumbs. Stir in the remaining ingredients.

3 Turn the hot fruit into a 4-cup ovenproof dish, spoon the crumble mixture over the top and bake in a preheated oven, 350°F, for 25–30 minutes or until golden-brown. Serve with custard or ice cream.

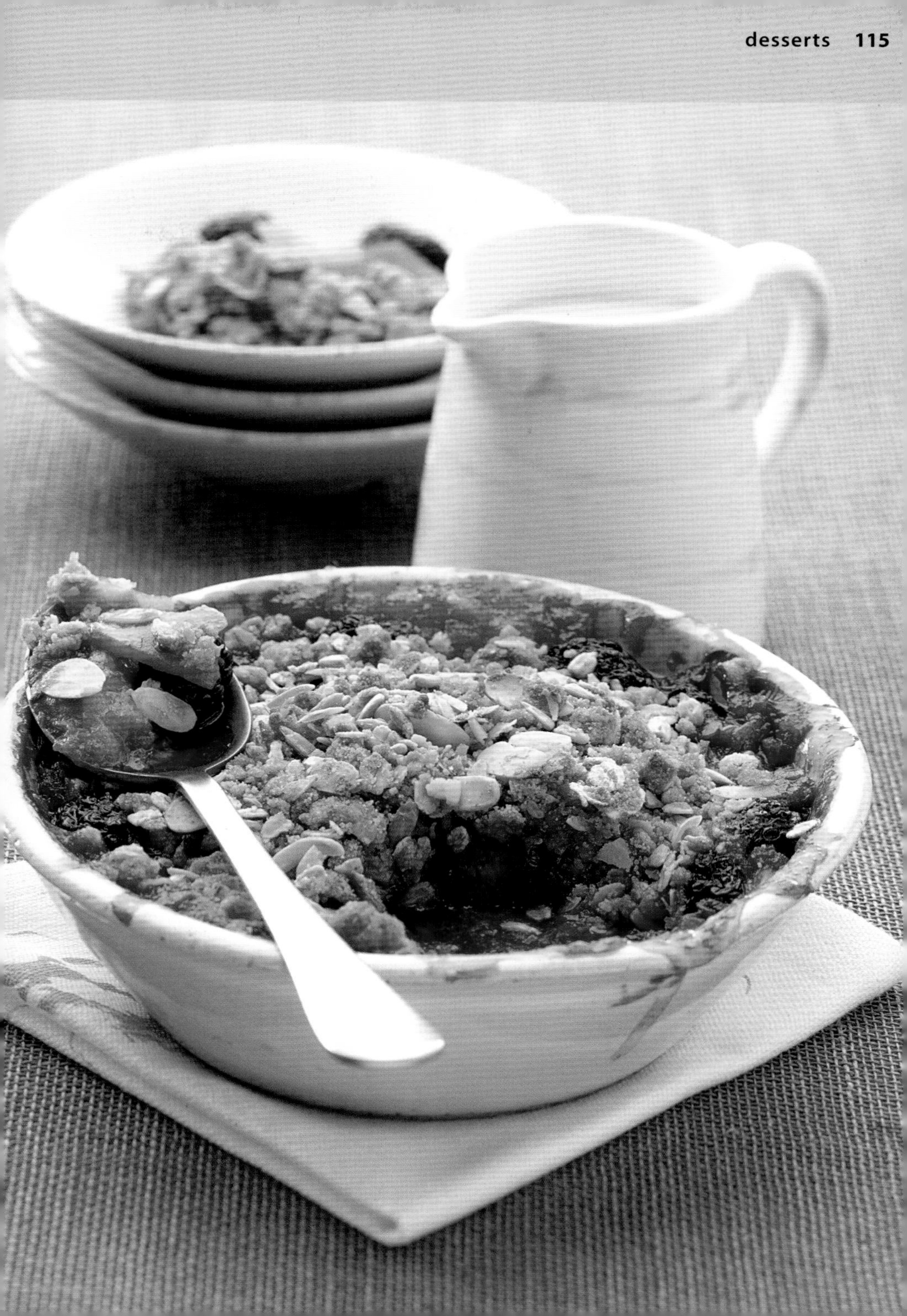

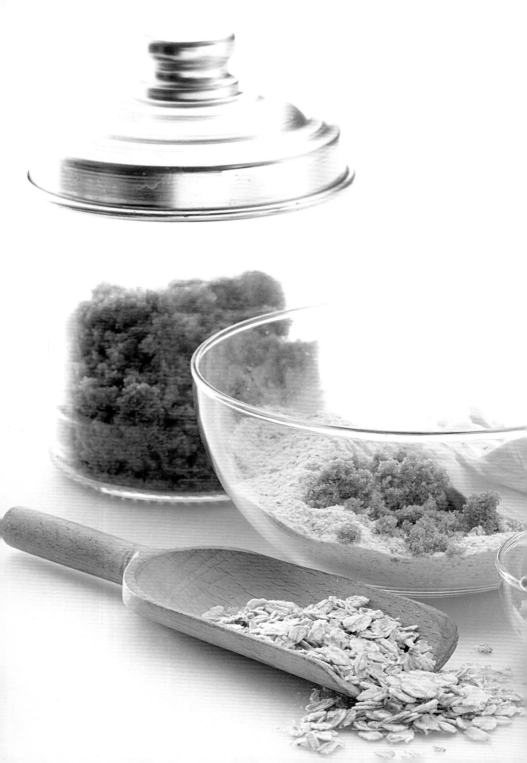

cakes and bakes

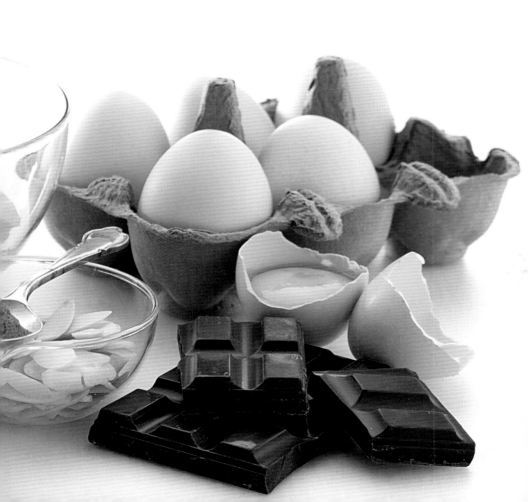

Nutrition
Wheat free, gluten free
Kcals 327
Fat 14 g
Saturated fat 1 g
Sodium 166 mg
Fiber 3 g

Preparation time
30 minutes, plus
cooling
Cooking time
15 minutes
Serves
8

 NUTRITIONAL TIP
If you are allergic to nuts but not wheat
or gluten, then fold in 1 cup sifted all-
purpose flour instead. Check the canned
cherries and cream cheese are gluten free.

cherry and orange roulade

Just because you may be intolerant to wheat flour doesn't mean that you must avoid
cakes. This wheat-free roulade uses ground almonds instead.

5 large eggs, separated

**1 cup superfine sugar, plus
extra for dusting**

1 cup ground almonds

grated zest of 1½ oranges

⅓ cup slivered almonds

1¼ cups lowfat cream cheese

**14 oz can stoned cherries,
drained**

a few fresh cherries (optional)

1 Put the egg yolks and ¾ cup sugar in a large bowl set over
a saucepan of simmering water. Beat until light and pale.
Take the bowl off the saucepan and gently fold in the ground
almonds and the zest from 1 orange.

2 Put the egg whites in a separate bowl and beat until stiff,
moist-looking peaks form. Fold a large spoonful into the yolk
mixture to loosen it slightly, then gently fold in the rest.

3 Grease and line a 9 x 12 inch baking pan with a piece of
nonstick parchment paper. Make diagonal cuts into the
corners of the paper, then press it into the pan. Pour in the
mixture and ease it into the corners. Sprinkle with the
slivered almonds and bake in a preheated oven, 350°F, for
15 minutes until the roulade is well risen and the top feels
spongy. Remove from the oven and allow to cool.

4 Beat the cream cheese with the remaining orange zest and
half the remaining sugar. Put a large piece of parchment
paper on the work surface, dust it with the remaining sugar
and turn the roulade out on it. Remove the lining paper.

5 Spread the cream cheese mixture over the top, then
sprinkle with the cherries. Roll up the roulade, starting from
the short edge, using the paper to help. Transfer to a serving
plate, remove the paper and cut into thick slices to serve.

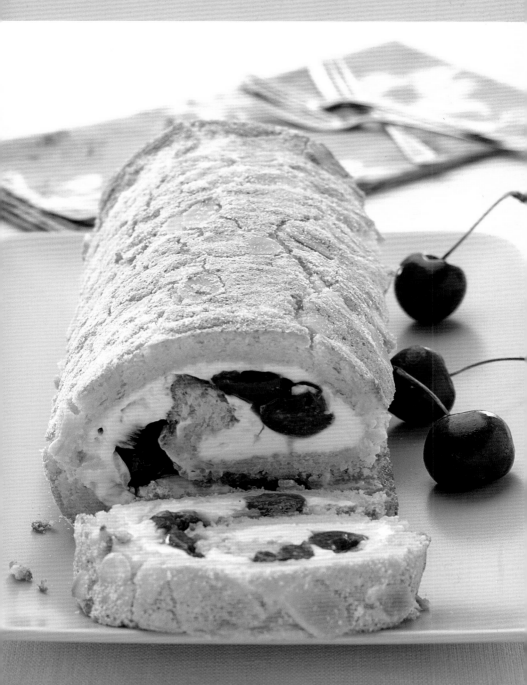

Nutrition

Low fiber

Kcals 66

Fat 3 g

Saturated fat 1 g

Sodium 69 mg

Fiber 1 g

Preparation time

20 minutes

Cooking time

10 minutes

Makes

24 cookies

NUTRITIONAL TIP

For a dairy-free version, use soy margarine and unsweetened soy milk instead of the lowfat spread and dairy milk. You will also need to omit the chocolate topping.

chocolate cinnamon cookies

Lower in fat and higher in fiber than most shop-bought cookies, these crumbly cookies are drizzled with a little chocolate for those moments when you crave something sweet.

1½ cups whole-wheat flour

2 teaspoons baking powder

1 teaspoon ground cinnamon

⅓ cup medium oatmeal

½ cup reduced-fat spread

3 tablespoons soft dark brown sugar

3 tablespoons lowfat milk

2 oz dark chocolate

1 Put the flour, baking powder, cinnamon, and oatmeal into a bowl. Add the spread and blend with fingertips until the mixture resembles fine bread crumbs.

2 Stir in the sugar, add the milk and mix to a soft but not sticky dough.

3 Knead lightly, then roll out on a lightly floured surface to ¼ inch thick. Cut out 2½ inch rounds with a fluted or plain cookie cutter. Transfer the cookies to an oiled baking sheet, then knead and re-roll the trimmings until all the mixture is used. Prick the cookies with a fork, then bake in a preheated oven, 400°F, for 10 minutes or until browned. Allow to cool.

4 Melt the chocolate in a bowl set over a pan of gently simmering water. Drizzle or pipe squiggly lines of chocolate from a spoon over the top of the cookies. Leave to harden for 20 minutes, then serve. The cookies will keep for up to 5 days in an airtight container.

Nutrition

Dairy free

Kcals 194

Fat 7 g

Saturated fat 2 g

Sodium 157 mg

Fiber 3 g

Preparation time

25 minutes

Cooking time

30–35 minutes

Makes

16 squares

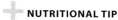 **NUTRITIONAL TIP**

To lower the level of fiber, use white flour rather than a mix of white and brown and omit the seeds on top. If you are not avoiding dairy products, use reduced-fat spread and lowfat cows' milk instead of the soy products.

banana and fig gingerbread

This moist, golden gingerbread is flecked with naturally sweet bananas and chopped dried figs, so that only syrup has been added to the cake rather than the more usual mix of syrup and sugar. This cake keeps well in an airtight container, so is ideal for adding to packed lunchboxes.

½ cup soy margarine

½ cup corn syrup

¾ cup figs, chopped

⅔ cup unsweetened soy milk

2 tablespoons chopped crystallized ginger

1 cup self-rising flour

1 cup plain whole-wheat flour

3 teaspoons ground ginger

1 teaspoon baking soda

2 ripe bananas, about 6 oz each with their skins on, peeled and mashed

2 eggs, beaten

2 tablespoons sunflower seeds (optional)

1 Put the margarine, syrup, figs, milk, and ginger in a saucepan and heat gently until the margarine has melted.

2 Mix all the dry ingredients together in a bowl. Beat the eggs in a second small bowl.

3 Take the saucepan off the heat, then mix in the bananas and dry ingredients with a wooden spoon. Gradually beat in the eggs.

4 Grease and line an 8 inch square cake pan and pour the mixture into the pan. Sprinkle with the seeds (if used) and bake in a preheated oven, 350°F, for 30–35 minutes until the cake is well risen and the top springs back when pressed with a fingertip. Allow the cake to cool in the pan.

5 Remove from the pan, peel off the lining paper and cut into 16 squares. Store in an airtight container for up to 7 days.

Nutrition

Wheat and gluten free, low fiber

Kcals 380

Fat 21 g

Saturated fat 11 g

Sodium 82 g

Fiber 2 g

Preparation time

40 minutes, plus

cooling

Cooking time

15–18 minutes

Serves

8

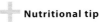 **Nutritional tip**

Choose chocolate that is 70 percent cocoa solids, as it should be completely wheat free and gluten free, but always check the label.

chocolate and raspberry layer cake

This wheat-free cake is perfect for a birthday celebration. Alternatively, serve it as a dessert with a drizzle of pureed raspberry sauce (see page 104). The cakes can be frozen on their own or fully assembled with the raspberries and chocolate curls.

7 oz bittersweet chocolate, chopped

6 eggs, separated

³/₄ cup superfine sugar, plus extra for dusting

2 tablespoons warm water

²/₃ cup whipping cream

1 cup Greek or whole milk yogurt

2 cups raspberries

chocolate curls, to decorate

1 Put the chocolate in a bowl set over a saucepan of gently simmering water and leave for 5 minutes until melted.

2 Lift the chocolate bowl off the pan, set a second large bowl on top of the water, add the egg yolks and sugar and beat for 5 minutes until very light and pale and the beaters leave a trail when lifted out of the mixture. Take the bowl off the pan and gently fold in the chocolate and measured warm water.

3 In a clean bowl beat the egg white until stiff but moist-looking peaks form. Fold a large spoonful into the yolks mixture to loosen it, then fold in the remainder.

4 Grease and line 2 round 8 inch layer pans and divide the mixture equally between them. Bake in a preheated oven, 350°F, for 15–18 minutes until well risen and the tops are crusty and cracked and softly set in the center. Remove from the oven. Allow to cool in the pans.

5 Whip the cream until it holds its shape, then fold in the yogurt. Turn out the cakes and put one on a serving plate. Top with half the cream mixture and half the raspberries. Add the second cake, the remaining cream and raspberries and then complete with a few chocolate curls. Cut into slices to serve.

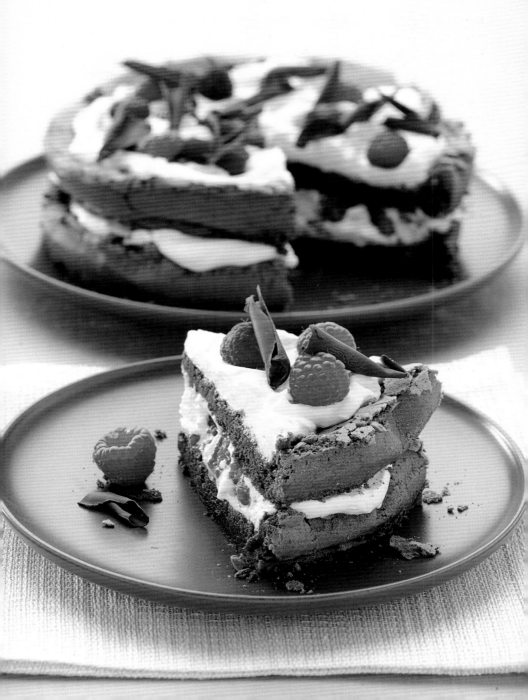

Nutrition

Wheat and gluten free, low fiber

Kcals 323

Fat 11 g

Saturated fat 3 g

Sodium 164 mg

Fiber 2 g

Preparation time

30 minutes

Cooking time

30–35 minutes

Serves

8

NUTRITIONAL TIP

White flour can be used if you are not on a wheat- or gluten-free diet. Use margarine to make this cake suitable for a dairy-free diet.

apple sauce cake

No one will guess that this cake is wheat free. Serve while it's still warm on its own or with a spoonful of reduced-fat sour cream or soy yogurt for a dairy-free alternative. Drizzled with custard, it doubles as a pudding.

2 cooking apples, each about 8 oz, cored, peeled, and thinly sliced

little lemon juice

2 cups wheat- and gluten-free white bread flour with natural gum

2½ teaspoons wheat- and gluten-free baking powder

1 teaspoon ground cinnamon

½ teaspoon ground ginger

¼ teaspoon grated nutmeg

3 eggs

⅔ cup reduced-fat spread

¾ cup superfine sugar

1 Put half the apple slices in a small saucepan with 2 tablespoons water, then cover and simmer for 5 minutes until pulpy. Put the remaining apple slices in a bowl of cold water with a little lemon juice.

2 Mix together the flour, baking powder, half the cinnamon, and all the ginger and nutmeg in a second bowl. Beat the eggs in a pitcher.

3 Cream the reduced-fat spread with ⅔ cup sugar in a bowl. Gradually mix alternate spoonfuls of egg and flour mix into the creamed mixture until both have been added and the mixture is smooth. Stir in the cooked apple.

4 Pour the mixture into a lightly oiled 9 inch springform cake pan and smooth the top. Drain the remaining apples well and arrange the slices in rings on top of the cake mixture. Sprinkle with the remaining sugar and cinnamon. Bake in a preheated oven, 350°F, for 35–40 minutes until well risen and a tester inserted into the center of the cake comes out cleanly.

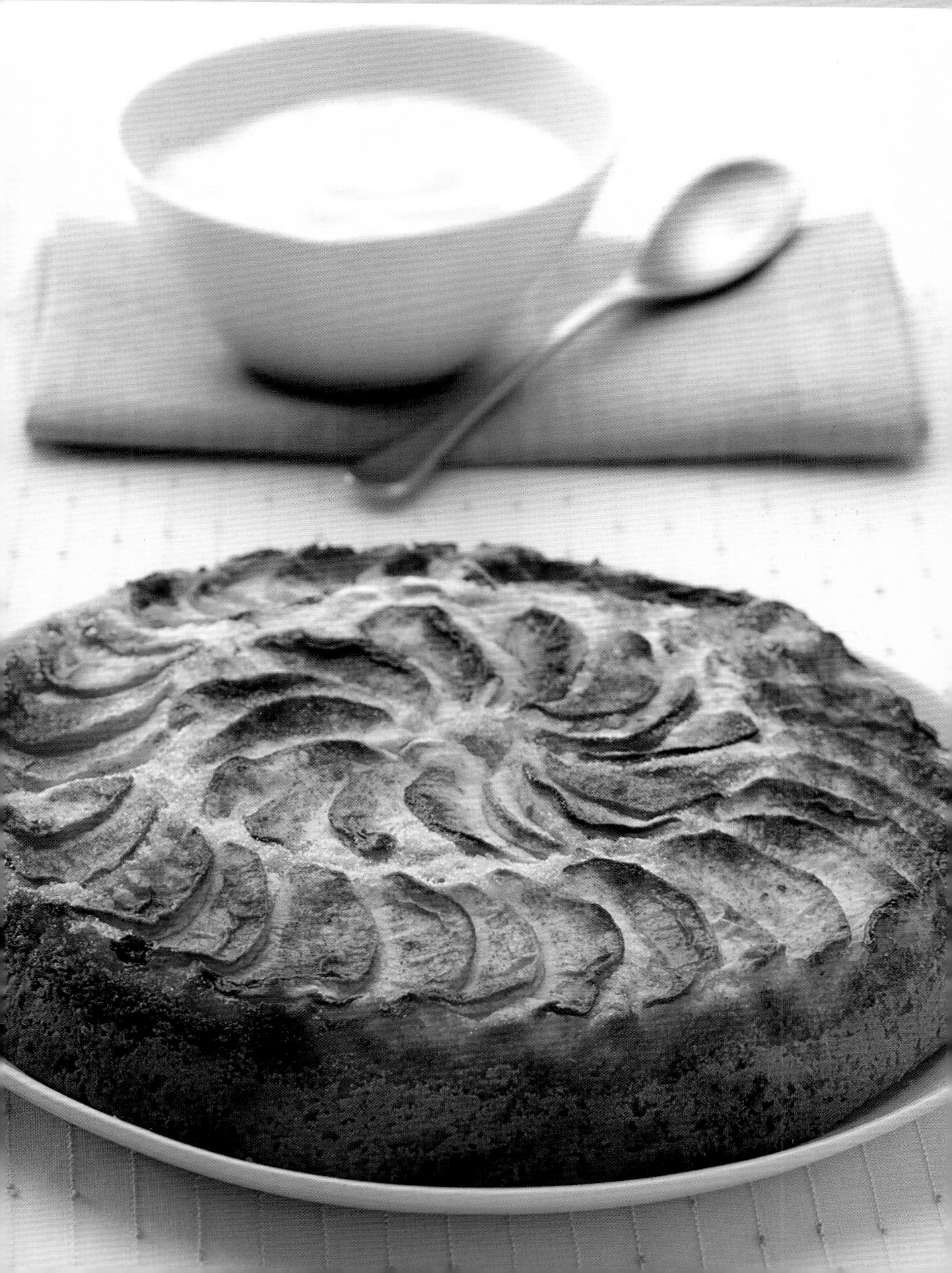

index

Useful contacts

Britain

IBS Network
Helpline: 0114 272 3253
www.ibsnetwork.org.uk
A national charity, providing the
only dedicated support in the UK
to people with IBS, helping them
and their families and carers to
manage their IBS and achieve
an improved quality of life. For
the fact sheet "IBS Information
and Advice" send a SAE to the
above address.

Allergy UK
Helpline: 01322 619898
www.allergyuk.org

British Dietetic Association
www.bda.uk.com
Access to an informative fact
sheet on a range of diet-related
issues written by registered
dietitians on their website.

British Society of Medical and
Dental Hypnosis
Tel: 07000 560 309
www.bsmdh.org
To search for a health professional
with expertise in hypnotherapy.

Dieticians Unlimited
www.dieticiansunlimited.co.uk
To search for a dietician with
expertise in IBS via their website.

Health Professions Council (HPC)
Tel: 020 7582 0866
www.hpc-uk.org
Check your dietitian is registered
by logging on to the HPC website.

Australia

Irritable Bowel Information and
Support Association of Australia
(IBIS Australia)
Tel: 0061 (0)7 3907 0527
www.ibis-australia.org

Dietitians Association of Australia
(DAA)
Tel: 0061 (0)2 6282 9555
www.daa.asn.au
You can find an Accredited
Practicing Dietitian (APD) who
has expertise in treating IBS.

Canada

IBS Association
www.ibsassociation.org

USA

IBS Association (IBSA)
www.ibsassociation.org

IBS Self-help Group (IBS Group)
www.ibsgroup.org

American Dietetic Association
www.eatright.org
Tel: 001 800 877 1600
You can find a registered nutrition
professional with expertise in IBS
through this site.

Acknowledgments

Tracy Parker would like to thank
Alex Riordan BSc (Hons) RD, Dr
David Preston, Dr Ed Stoner and
Helen Francis for their helpful
comments and advice.

Executive editor: Nicola Hill
Editor: Camilla Davis
Executive art editor:
    Darren Southern
Home economist: Sara Lewis
Designer: Colin Goody
Picture research: Jennifer Veall
Production: Nigel Reed

Picture credits

Special photography:
© **Octopus Publishing Group
Ltd**/William Lingwood

Other photograpy:
Corbis UK Ltd 10. **Getty
Images**/Pierre Bourrier 19.
**Octopus Publishing Group
Ltd**/Frank Adam 36 top; /Jean
Cazals 14; /Stephen Conroy 11, 17
top, 21 top, 26, 27; /David Jordan
35 bottom; /Sandra Lane 3 centre;
/William Lingwood 1, 2 left, 2
centre, 4–5, 13; /David Loftus 18;
/Neil Mersh 15, 23 top, 36 bottom;
/Peter Myers 31; /Lis Parsons 3, 23
bottom; /William Reavell 3 left, 20,
25, 33; /Craig Robertson 24;
/Russell Sadur 32; /Gareth
Sambidge 2 right, 34; /Simon
Smith, 18 top; /Ian Wallace 12, 21
bottom, 28, 36 centre.
Photolibrary 9. **Photodisc** 7.